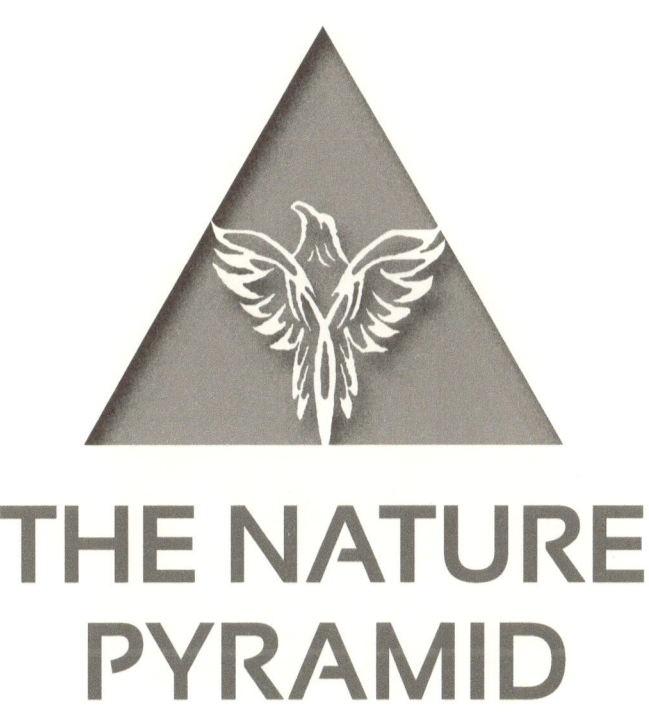

THE NATURE PYRAMID

Anthony James Canelo

ISBN: 1496078969

ISBN-13: 9781496078964

Library of Congress Control Number: 2014903932

CreateSpace Independent Publishing Platform

North Charleston, South Carolina

OTHER BOOKS BY ANTHONY CANELO

The Seven Fundamentals of Longevity

Marriage, Incarceration, Death, Religion, and Patience

Sleep: The Great Medicine

Folk Remedies for the Modern Age

Slowness Gives Wholeness

The Complete Compact Guide to Disaster Survival

The Revival of the Fittest: A Manual to Change the World

Revival of the Fittest: The Prime Material for Human Health and Wisdom

Self Determination: The Strategy for Mastering Addiction in America

TABLE OF CONTENTS

"Poor soul, the center of sinful earth, foiled by those rebel powers that thee array. Why dost thy pine within and suffer dirth, painting thy outward walls so costly gay? Why so large cost, having so short a lease, dost thou upon thy fading mansion spend? Shall worms, inheritors of this excess, eat up thy charge? Is this thy body's end? Then soul, live thou upon thy servant's loss, and let that pine to aggravate thy store buy terms divine in selling hours of dross within be fed, without be rich no more. So shalt thou feed on death, that feeds on men and, death once dead, there's no more dying then."

— William Shakespeare

INTRODUCTION

I wrote these twenty essays as introductions to my radio show. Afterward, I decided it was best to give longevity to my words in book form. My focus and message are about a connection with nature. I feel compelled to describe it in as many ways as I possibly can. This is my passion. I hope you enjoy the essays as much as I enjoyed writing them.

A very special thank you Sam Leibowitz of Talking Alternative Broadcasting; Vision NDNS; and my mother, Emily Canelo.

The following poem "It is That" I wrote for my radio show. It was inspired by my beautiful poet friend Andrew, the Ramtha School of Enlightenment, and the mystery that lives within.

IT IS THAT...

It is that song of the cosmos, or music of the spheres,
the Garden of Eden, of unnumbered years.
It is that whole brain of Brahman, illuminated mind,
the great self of old, before there was time.
The psychic brain, the god within,
sun and moon, will of the wind.
Deep sleep of Shiva, sole path of truth,
revelation of the self, the fountain of youth.
The great soul expressing the word and the law,
primordially joyful, unmasked, and raw.
It is that kingdom of heaven, in days of yore,
the Nebulae light, where the fire is born.
It is that creator of universes, the one true god,
life beyond time, every second, on.
It is that magic number one, from cradle to grave,
the epic of the Cristos, the ace of spades.
Running through potentials in eternities stride.
The dreamer has awakened, saddled to ride,
the river of time. It is that sacred channel,
electrified brains, great drums and rattles.
It is that missing link to that forever joy,
the sweet innocent girl and the humble boy.
It is that flavor that taste, that sound, that waist,
that created new life in its natural pace.
It is that hill and that sun.
It is the song of the one.

It is that shadow and truth.
It is the God inside you.
It is that fire of hope, the dance without death,
a raging river and morning's sweet breath.
It is all that I am, naked and blue,
that unnatural pain I must undo.
It is that alchemical marriage, beyond blood skin and bone,
that unmapped expression, alpha, omega, star seed, home.
It is that sacred room, life and sweet death,
it is what is is, between right and left,
betwixt lower and higher,
it sits eternally, internally wired.
It is that deaf man's poem, the serpent in the sky,
a great white silence, the all in all, AUM NAMAHA SHIVAI.
It is that mind inside the seven seals, the seven churches, the seven steps, the
seven heavens,
the seven bodies, the seven signs,
the seven chakras, the seven minds,
the seven symbols, the seven degrees,
the seven spheres, and the seven seas.
For there are more things in heaven and Earth that are dreamt of in your
philosophy. Once death has died life will spring anew, Horatio, anew.
It is that intelligent design with a lawless mind, through perfected desire,
discovers truth so sublime and unmired, as to collide with your soul,
where peace is profound and pain never seen,
its far past the visions in your wildest dreams.
It is the years gone by, it is that unknown caller,
laughter, jewels, and riches, poverty and squalor.
It is the infrared body, the light body, the ultraviolet blue body, the x-ray
body, the golden section.
It is the answer to your greatest question.

It is the moment, the mirror, the forever love of freedom.
It is the shadow world, the dark matter, the nether world, the ether.
It is that ancient sound inside the sun that they call point zero…or the one.
It is the void. It is the stillness behind the logos, the hologram of the Helios.
It is the quantum observer or the unified field,
the unseen movements, the tree of life, the real.
You can hear about it now or die into it later.
It is that light of god, the stain glass window.
It is "bountis ad infinitum," of which there is none greater.
It is the quintessence, seventh heaven, irreproachably aware.
Each is their director sitting in their director's chair.
It is that something out of nothing, from the center of a pearl.
The line and the curve, the foundations of the world.
It is that footstep in the sand, the philosopher's stone
that in the light of all eternity beckons to the unknown.
It is that breath of life that flows next to me.
It is the light of truth. It is that spiritual ecstasy.
Like a pearl in the sand, from dawn until dusk,
a rose in spring, the pure eyes you can trust,
they make no disguises, having left them behind,
and sing to the night, until the end of all time.

I DESERVE TO BE
THE BEST I CAN BE

"What if you could wake up before a fire? What if we didn't need GPS to get us to the hospital in an emergency? What if we didn't need somebody telling us what is unhealthy and healthy, we just knew? What if you could conveniently avoid paying taxes and sense the IRS coming from hundreds of miles away? What if you could track down a good job, or for that matter a decent relationship, with your nose like a bloodhound? All of these natural qualities are potentials for humankind. However, today few people can recognize evolution under the hoods of their own cars, in their pantries, or especially in their lives."

There is a feeling that arises in people, usually later in life, that encourages them to find meaning in their lives. It's often called a midlife crisis. It makes people tear off their goggles and often causes a complete lifestyle reversal. What direction do they reverse toward? Nature. This event that we call a "personal crisis" has actually happened to people throughout history. Only recently with the Internet, cinema, and coffee-table conversation have we begun to learn just how common it is. It's perfectly natural. What's so natural about it? Perhaps for the first time people recognized vacuums in themselves. Nature, it is said, abhors a vacuum and struggles to fill a void. Unfortunately, this sort of pivotal desire is mocked and passed off as weakness in modern society. In the West we are empowered by the computers, phones, movies, games, and events that disguise the void inside us and serve as incompatible fulfillments that we begin to crave.

I once read a story about an amazing man named Luther Burbank. Luther Burbank was responsible for advancing the science of agriculture almost twenty-five years ahead of his time. Burbank coined the terms "hybridizing" and "burbanking" and was a boon to the U.S. Department of Agriculture in the 1920s. His story is unbelievable. At the tail end of his incredible career, he was called a charlatan for growing human-sized watermelons, raising orchards of plum trees in only a couple of years, and consistently developing new species of plants. Then an earthquake hit California, and its epicenter was close to Burbank's country home and greenhouse. The surrounding area was devastated, but his property remained undamaged—not a broken window or a fallen tree. Naturally, this attracted attention from the newspaper. Reporters flocked to his property and called it another of his, quote, "miracles." They wanted to know his secret. He responded to the reporters quite frankly, with a statement I will personally never forget: "My secret," he said, "is a rapid elimination of nonessentials."

Isn't that the ticket?

Many would call a midlife crisis an omen or a curse. I call it a sign of greatness. The question is, what is this emptiness all about, and how can we use it? The answer varies with each individual. However, there is strong evidence pointing in the direction of nature, and we will talk about what that evidence looks like. When I use the word *nature*, I'm not just talking about cirrus clouds, butterflies, and maple syrup. I'm actually talking about an evolving quality, an interior set of principles and motives influencing how we behave and how we live every moment common to all life. I'm talking about an instinct, an intelligence. This process has been called "evolution" by Charles Darwin or "morphology" by Johann Goethe, and there are many controversial interpretations surrounding these ideas, but when we're faced with a personal crisis—a depression or a deep well of emptiness—how does evolution appear in life? If you're not going to analyze fruit flies under a microscope or speak sign language with a gorilla, what does evolution look like in your nine-to-five everyday life?

Nature is an evolving quality. What if nature was rapping at your door right now? Have you ever watched domesticated dogs chew grass when they get sick? Have you ever seen salmon travel upstream to lay their eggs in the exact same spot where they were born, after months of traveling the ocean? Birds have been known to do the same thing. Bears have been observed to wake from hibernation before major earthquakes. Sharks, according to a 2008 research study by Michelle Heupel of Mote Marine Laboratory, can actually detect hurricanes from hundreds of miles away and conveniently avoid them. What if you could wake up before a fire? What if we didn't need GPS to get us to the hospital in an emergency? What if we didn't need somebody telling us what is unhealthy and healthy, we just knew? What if you could conveniently avoid paying taxes and sense the IRS coming from hundreds of miles away? What if you could track down a good job, or for that matter a decent relationship, with your nose like a bloodhound? All of these natural qualities are potentials for humankind. However, today few people can recognize evolution under the hoods of their own cars, in their pantries, or especially, in their lives. If you have evolution going on in your life, wouldn't it be nice to give yourself some due credit? Where is it?

Okay, I'll tell you. Have you realized that a small handful of inventors created the Industrial Revolution and that the entire consumer corporate world owes an uncountable debt to twelve men?

- Cyrus Fiel for the transatlantic cable
- Samuel Morse for the telegraph
- Robert Fulton for the steamboat
- Eli Whitney for the cotton gin
- Rupert Diesel for the diesel engine
- Nikola Tesla for the induction motor
- Elias Howe for the sewing machine
- Thomas Edison for the phonograph and the light bulb
- Alexander Graham Bell for the telephone
- Henry Ford for the large-scale moving assembly line

I forgot George Washington Carver for improved peanut butter and many other things. Without Mr. Diesel there would be no diesel. Without Elias and Whitney we'd be wearing very interesting clothes. Without Edison and Graham Bell, there'd be no *Revival of the Fittest Radio Hour.* Are we more evolved because of them? No. Yet who among all of these inventors was comfortable with the question of the vacuum, the void in their own life? They discovered necessity because they were incredibly curious. Each of them refused to accept distraction and was never comfortable with living in the status quo. Today we owe it all to them. That's what made these people great. What do they have in common? Yes, they were lovers of their own kind, but they were also lovers of nature. We live in a country where people have the chance to break the Gordian knot of survival and evolve, contribute, share their own greatness with the world if at all possible. Were these people evolving? You can absolutely bet they were.

George Washington Carver once said, "Anything will give up its secrets if you love it enough. Not only have I found that when I talk to the little flower or the little peanut, they will give up their secrets, but I have found that when I silently commune with people they give up their secrets also, if you love them enough." Who in their right mind would disagree with me when I say that George Washington Carver was a lover of nature? Albert Einstein said, "Nothing will benefit human health and increase the chances of survival of life on Earth as much as the evolution to a vegetarian diet." Who in their right mind would disagree if I said Albert Einstein took excellent care of his physical health? Nikola Tesla was known for his feats of athleticism and self-imposed periods of fasting and meditation that sometimes lasted two or three days. He even claimed that for most of his life he never deviated one pound in his weight! In his autobiography he claimed to be able to digest cobblestones. With that guy, one never knows.

Johann Goethe once said there are "Nine requisites for contented living: Health enough to make work a pleasure. Wealth enough to support your needs. Strength to battle with difficulties and overcome them. Grace enough to confess your sins and forsake them. Patience enough to toil until some good is accomplished. Charity enough to see some good in your neighbor. Love enough to move you to be useful and helpful to others. Faith enough to make real the things of God. Hope enough to remove all anxious fears concerning the future." It all starts with *health*. Someone once said that Goethe had an IQ of 210. Regardless, health was clearly a priority in his life. I sense that there is a great connection to nature in his words.

So we have a number of people who have essentially created our world for us and who also were evolving nature lovers. Then we have the champion medical doctors and specialists such as Emanuel Revici, Weston A. Price, Carey Reams, Nicholas Gonzalez, Gary Null, Paul C. Bragg, Majid Ali, Brian Clement, and Maynard Murray—students of nature who were and are still dedicated to the healing work. In fact, I'm going to read you a list of the many great humanitarians, artists, philosophers, writers, scientists, and statesmen who were or are vegetarians, also known for their intense love of nature:

Pythagoras	Henry David Thoreau
Plato	Richard Wagner
Arthur Schopenhauer	Jean Rousseau
Albert Schweitzer	François Voltaire
Albert Einstein	Benjamin Franklin
Mahatma Gandhi	Charles Darwin
Rabindranath Tagore	Ralph Emerson
Bob Dylan	Percy Bysshe Shelley
Isaac Newton	George Bernard Shaw
William Shakespeare	Louisa May Alcott

This is not to suggest that vegetarians are superior or more spiritual than the rest of humanity. However, it does underscore the fact that many people of integrity, intelligence, and achievement have adopted a much more substantial connection to nature.

Tomorrow morning, remind yourself: "I deserve to be the best that I can be." Look at this; is this the hidden secret of genius—examining how you eat, what you drink, how you feel, how you breathe, how you sleep, and your level of physical fitness? Is it a connection to nature? Do you think this is in any way strange? Perhaps there really is more in heaven and Earth than is dreamt of in your philosophy, Horatio. Look at the actors who are charming, talented, and nature lovers: Tom Hanks, Leonardo DiCaprio, Cameron Diaz, Salma Hayak, and so many others. My point is, in a crisis of emptiness, there is a void. The challenge is fill it with an original mind that can make us great people, great children, or great teachers. The past is the past. Your life, if it is a changing life, can become a rhapsody of passion, love, and creative impulse. Take a deep breath.

Did you know that deep sea divers train for months to reach peak physical condition so that they can see the bottom of the ocean for themselves? Sailors used to eat lemons to maintain their vitamin C levels and keep scurvy away. Astronauts train underwater, lift weights, eat a healthy diet, and maintain a regular sleep cycle. What do *they* get to see? What about Ernest Shackleton, the first man to explore the South Pole? Don't you think he took care of his health as well? When he got there, he said, "We had seen God in his splendors, heard the text that nature renders, we had reached the naked soul of man." Every great explorer, artist, genius, and inventor comes up against this interior vacuum, this void. The world may think it's strange that they seek the secrets of nature, but what does the world know? Just go for it. When others laugh, enjoy it. Without that wonderful elixir of creativity, most of life is predictable. You deserve to be the best that you can be, because it's in you to do so. You can be your own personal sailor. Somebody's on the phone, and it's you. Find that legendary fulfillment, because anything will give up its secrets if you love it enough.

THE GREAT
QUESTIONS

"Your Body is your Private Property."

When I sense that people are searching for help, I like to ask them four questions:

1. What is the smallest thing you can do that would help create the largest shift in your life?

2. What is the largest thing you can do that would create the most insignificant shift in your life?

3. Which unhealthy habit could you cease that would yield the smallest real effect on your life?

4. What is the simplest, smallest thing you could stop doing that would bring on the most tremendously powerful impact for the good in your own life?

In other words, how insightful are you into your resistance to progressive change? Tell me about your weakest links. Share with me the extent of your knowledge and experience. Help me understand the terrain of your mind.

I prefer not to be a victim of the outdated traditions of a historically corrupt system. I prefer to live as a sovereign in my own life—source my own food and water, protect myself, and give myself plenty of open space with land and shelter. I imagine everyone shares a part of this dream in some way. History is replete with cycles. Through time people have come together into cities for the causes of trade, religion, war, limited resources, and so on. Then people disperse throughout the land for many of the same reasons. At a later date, they come together again. Clearly, we are at a tail end in this repeating pattern of self-reliance. Who wants to fill their minds with *Who Wants to be a Millionaire?*, the televised survival realities, violence, drugs, fame, sex, and infamy, without any morals or reason for living? These things pull us closer to a completely dependent end of the spectrum. All my life I have heard, "History is replete with cycles. However, it is the wise person that seeks to break free from these cycles." What other cycles are we are trying to break free from, other than the cycles of private property and corporate government ownership or eminent domain? In this country there are cycles of poverty and war that are as reliable as the weather. There are predictable cycles of mass incarceration. There are financial cycles. There are cycles of leadership and political uprising that are carefully suppressed every four years by events we call "elections" that also contain smaller cycles of fraud. Why do I use private property and collective ownership as a metaphor? Because your body is your *private property.* John Locke was absolutely correct when he said that private property is a *natural* right. Private property is the basis of all subsequent freedoms. If people treated their bodies half as well as they treat their houses or homes, we would be living in a brave new world.

Imagine what President Obama would say to the first question, "What is the smallest thing you can do that would help create the largest shift in your life?" Would he speak against Citizens United or the drone wars? What about the largest thing you can do that would create the most insignificant shift in your life? Perhaps he would plug his new health care regime. What about the simplest, smallest thing you could stop doing that would bring on the most tremendously powerful impact for the good in your own life? Perhaps he would stop smoking. How would Hillary answer these questions? How many ways has she wasted her time in power? Let's consider a crack addict from Manhattan. We'll call him Leon. How would Leon answer that first question? Perhaps he would say, "Get myself into a shelter." The answers change with one's station, obviously. Imagine Leon won the lottery and bought himself a boat to sail around the world. That could be the largest thing yielding no true benefit, of course—because Leon is still smoking crack. (No offense to any people named Leon from Manhattan who currently smoke crack.)

Aren't these questions delicious? If confronted with enough truth, you begin to reach for that rare diamond called "common sense." These questions are meant to exercise common sense. What *is* common sense? It is the ability to distill large amounts of information very quickly. Why not get to the root, the seed of your personal and health concerns? Here are the factors that influence your health the most: You are what you eat. You are what you think. You are how you breathe. You are what you drink. You are how you move. You are what you feel. All of these will keep your connection to nature real, fortified, and pure. You are the lord or lady of your own life. That's you. You.

I once asked, "How may I serve?" I knew it was in me to do what I'm doing now. My thirst for reason and knowledge comes second nature. Throughout history people have been murdered or publicly rebuked for asking too many questions, from Socrates to Jesus to Howard Zinn. Why? When you ask yourself a question, you open up a door of inquiry. The question allows us to think for ourselves. What are the most profound questions? "Who am I?" "What am I?" "What is my objective here?" Where are the dangerous questions, the questions people are afraid to ask? Those are the questions that wring out your internal organs as though they were a piece of wet cloth. I'd like to ask you some questions. What do you think about the 1 billion people around the world who smoke cigarettes daily? Did you know that people who smoke cigarettes daily account for 50 percent of all the people with mental illness in our country? How do you feel about that? Did you know alcohol is the most widely used drug in the world and that 28 million children around the country are living with an alcoholic adult? No other form of disability costs individuals, employers, and governments more money in treatment, injuries, reduced worker productivity, and property damage than alcoholism. What do you really think about that? Now, who is perpetuating and perpetrating all of this? Isn't *that* an excellent question?

What do you think about the 60 percent of adults who do not engage in any vigorous exercise (that is, exercise that requires heavy breathing and sweating)? What do you think about the fact that people who don't exercise are more likely to develop cancer, diabetes, osteoporosis, hypertension, and metabolic syndrome? Six out of ten college students use drugs.[1] One out of every four Americans is said to be suffering from a mental illness.[2] One out of every seventeen people is said to have a serious mental illness. Twenty million women and ten million men suffer from a significant eating disorder sometime in their lives.[3]

---

[1] Hales, Dianne. *An Invitation to Health,* 15th ed. Stamford: Cenage Learning, 2012.

[2] National Institute of Mental Health. The Numbers Count: Mental Disorders in America. Available from: http://www.nimh.nih.gov/health/publications/the-numbers-count-mental-disorders-in-america/index.shtml.

[3] National Institute of Mental Health. What Are Eating Disorders? 2011. Available from: http://www.nimh.nih.gov/health/publications/eating-disorders/index.shtml

In the past two decades, virtually all mental health statistics have been on the rise.

Here's the big question: What is the most appropriate step you can make to improve your own quality of life? Someone at *Forbes* magazine once asked themselves a truly excellent question: What are the most preventable causes of death in this country? They found that smoking, alcohol, toxic lifestyles, sexually transmitted diseases, lack of nutrition, lack of exercise, and drugs encompassed the answer. I read the article and wrote a book on it called *Self Determination*. I'm not on the air to sell my book to you, however; I'm here to query your mind a little more.

What does the world really want? Does the world want to be saved or be comfortable? Does it want to simply survive? In lieu of the statistics I've mentioned, perhaps that is the case. We are struggling to survive. You can catch a fish and feed a family, and they will be comfortable for a night, or you can teach a family how to fish and save them. However, not everyone is excited to learn or willing to admit that they haven't learned yet how to fish.

A healer heals with the gentlest persuasion, a kind of persuasion that can pacify the edge of your comfort zone. That's why healers ask questions, and that is why someone who is trying to fix him- or herself needs to start with the questions. The next time you visit a hospital, ask them to check how hydrated your body is. Ask them to check you bone mass, your body fat, and your blood pressure. Ask them about prevention. Ask them about diet and exercise. Ask them questions. That's how things are going to change. Open your own mouth in the mirror and take a look at your own tongue. Is it white, red, pale, scratched? Look into purchasing a book on iridology and then look into your eyes.

Do you know your own bone mass or your hydration level? Don't you think that is a fabulous question? "How are my bones doing?" A wise man once said "The first casualty of war is truth." Even if it takes you many attempts to discover your truth, so what? Maybe it's better to avoid excess in all things and begin healing from scratch. All you have to do is ask the questions. This is the kind of world where such things are possible, and the answers are out there.

HEALTH & CULTURE

"The problem is this; the alternative talk became rigid and refused to acknowledge its wholeness. It's just another way to say divide and conquer."

"About 100 years ago, the various groups that composed our health care system (homeopathic doctors, eclectic physicians, osteopaths, Western herbalists, etc.) did not know how to get along with each other either. They constantly fought and argued over silly things. This led to their undoing. They might have been able to see eye to eye with the fundamental concepts of natural healing provided to them by Avicenna, Galen, and Hippocrates. However, there came a day when a wealthy, politically powerful entity named the American Medical Association effectively seized control of America's health care through its own government!"

There are as many definitions of a "healthy lifestyle" as there are countries and tribes across the world. In a sense, there have to be. Every environment has limited resources from which to eat, exercise, and lead a long, healthy life. For Eskimos, horse racing and tropical fruit salads were out of the question. However, the Eskimos learned how to fish and ride dogsleds and eventually dance on ice. These very pleasant activities became synonymous with a healthy lifestyle. Native Hawaiians never made the long, nomadic treks across continents searching for food. With no foreign armies attacking them and ocean on all sides, the Hawaiians quite naturally led slow lives. Slowness and patience are a few of the famed virtues of "healthy" Hawaiian living. It's called Lomi Lomi. With every culture comes a culturally specific definition of a healthy lifestyle, and our culture is no exception.

There is a beautiful and funny story written by Franz Kafka called *A Hunger Artist*. It begins, "During these last decades the interest in professional fasting has markedly diminished. It used to pay very well to stage such great performances under one's own management, but today that is quite impossible." The hunger artist is a professional fasting artist who locks himself in a cage on stage in front of hordes of spectators. The artist has an agent who takes him across Europe to give his forty-day shows, but eventually public interest diminishes, so he decides to join a circus. The fasting artist eventually loses his good health, and the story has a great ending that I won't tell you. Essentially the fasting artist was living for the opinions of other people, his culture, and his personal creed. You can imagine the type of culture that promotes this type of fundamentally unnatural body and self image, can't you? If you think about it, you could easily put a cigarette smoker, a drug addict, or an alcoholic in a cage, and it would all serve to illustrate the damaging effects of public opinion on human health. Imagine that.

Maybe we should stop here and say that a healthy lifestyle is only relative to one's own culture. I personally think that would make no sense at all; we all have a common denominator, and that is the ground called nature. Now we can examine how a greater alignment with nature impacts health. Check out Japan, Switzerland, Iceland, or Germany.[4] Look at the longest-lived tribes of Armenia, Tibet, southern Russia, or

---

[4] WHO 2013 Life Expectancy

South America. So many of the longest-lived people in the world live in simple agricultural environments without the benefits of television, war, rush-hour traffic, or drugs. Life expectancy in Japan is usually one of the highest in the world, dwarfing American life expectancy. How does health influence culture? Well, the Japanese are renowned for their cultural exactness and economic productivity. A couple of years ago you could find ginger and burdock root on the menu in a Tokyo McDonalds. No kidding. Burdock root and ginger are incredible roots for healing and health maintenance.

The World Health Organization once reported that 75 percent of all people in the world are under some form of natural health care. That is not to say that everyone on a natural health care plan is healthy and long lived; there are millions in the dirty slums of Africa and southern India without the benefit of good hygiene and adequate sleep. Nonetheless, if you were to pick a horse in the Grand Prix of life expectancy, I would suggest you bet your gold, silver, and bronze on those countries that are holding fast to their connection to nature. What is a connection to nature? It comprises how well you sleep, how deeply you breathe, how hydrated you are, your diet, your fitness level, and whether you are of sound mind. Your connection to nature can also be severed by a lack of sensory stimulation, such as sunlight, grounding, fresh air, clean water for hygiene, and unpolluted foods.

If somebody on the other side of town is 118 years old, wouldn't you like to know what they might recommend as far as diet, lifestyle, and connection to nature? If a 118-year-old woman told you to drink at least one liter of water every morning before you ate anything, would you follow her instructions? Imagine you are shaking hands with that woman, and her name is "Japan." Better yet, let's imagine her name is "Madam Cuba." As Ms. or Mr. America, you would take heed to what she recommends. You would tell your family back home. America in 2013 was thirty-fifth in the world for life expectancy. Up ahead, near the front of the race, Hong Kong came in fifth, Japan came in second, Iceland came in seventh, Italy came in eighth place, Canada came in twelfth, Israel came in fourteenth, and Monaco came in first. According to the international ranking of countries in the Organisation for Economic Co-operation and Development, American students are performing at a mediocre level. America incarcerates more of its citizens than any other nation in the world. I'm not claiming to make a direct correlation between health and culture, but, if I were you, I would listen to that 118-year-old woman, because she might know a thing or two.

Where did natural health care truly begin? Most likely, it began in a valley in Ethiopia, the cradle of humanity, the place from which we all came. For the West, health care began with a Roman doctor surgeon named Pedanius Dioscorides. Dioscorides compiled the first truly comprehensive reference for medicinal plants in nature; *De Materia Medica* was produced in the first century and has been quoted and copied to this day. It is the prototype and platform for all herbal pharmacopoeias that have followed. Galen was another legendary physician and writer who discovered that arteries carry blood, not air. He added to the knowledge of the brain, spinal cord, nerves, and pulse, and his teachings dominated medical thought for fifteen hundred years. Herbal preparations are still called Galenic preparations. Many have said that if Galen were to visit our world today, he would laugh at the water supplies of many of our cities compared with the magnificent aqueducts of Rome. In communities with imperfect drainage or poor sanitation, he could serve as a sanitation expert. He could walk to the fields to prepare healing gargles, snuffs, salves, poultices, suppositories, fumigants, enemas, plasters, and inhalations like any good doctor of his day; he would marvel at our arrogance and our blatant detachment from the natural world. Then there is Hippocrates. Hippocrates was a renown advocate for the healing power of nature— the *vis medicatrix naturae*—in the form of diet and hygiene. He taught that medicine should add the patient's strength during crisis, never deplete it. The phrase *primum non nocere* means "First, do no harm," and is part of the Hippocratic Oath taken by all physicians in this country. Hippocrates had a few other famous sayings, one being "Let thy food be thy medicine and thy medicine by the food," and another, "Natural forces within us are the true healers of disease."

Where does this leave us? Today nature schools are popping up across America. Honest people are bending their limbs and planting seeds. People are eating local and avoiding polluted foods; they are composting, going solar, driving electric, and purifying their water. People are fiercely questioning whether it is safe and correct to live by the status quo or to accept what the governing body says about this or that. Thanks to the Internet, the average eighteen-year-old is exposed to almost twelve times the amount of information than their counterparts were back in 1960. The problem is, the alternative talk became rigid and refused to acknowledge its wholeness. It's just another way to say divide and conquer.

About 100 years ago, the various groups that composed our health care system (homeopathic doctors, eclectic physicians, osteopaths, Western herbalists, etc.) did not know how to get along with each other either. They constantly fought and argued over silly things. This led to their undoing. They might have been able to see eye to eye with the fundamental concepts of natural healing provided to them by Avicenna, Galen, and Hippocrates. However, there came a day when a wealthy, politically powerful entity named the American Medical

Association effectively seized control of America's health care through its own government! If you're trying to explore and fortify your connection to nature, and you are like most people, then you're reading all the blogs and websites you can find that attempt to distill the incredible amounts of information you've been given. The way I see it, that's "info overload," and that is the reason we—*Revival of the Fittest Radio*—are on the job.

No matter how complex and knowledgeable we are as a culture, it does nobody any good to lose track of common sense. What is common sense? Common sense allows us to process lots of information in a short period of time. I'm going to ask you four questions that I have asked every one of my guests at the Phoenix Institute of Holistic Health:

1. What is the smallest thing you can do that would help create the largest shift in your life?

2. What is the largest thing you can do that would create the most insignificant shift in your life?

3. Which unhealthy habit could you cease that would yield the smallest real effect on your life?

4. What is the simplest, smallest thing you could stop doing that would bring on the most tremendously powerful impact for the good in your own life?

Don't answer yet. I would rather you think about it for a minute. Perhaps you could start a conversation with friends. I've only asked you because I've learned to ask this of myself, and when it comes to healing and health, the answer that is most beautiful to me is "A connection to nature." My friends, that includes your level of fitness, hydration, nutrition, respiration, restfulness, and inspiration.

Why would you ever want to strengthen your connection with nature? Because it can give you real human quality, real alternatives. My show is about health and culture, real alternatives, and what you can do to help yourself survive and thrive.

RELATIONSHIPS & CREATIONSHIPS

"How do we screen for sexually transmitted relationship issues? I'm going to help you with that. Find a pen and write these words down: vulnerophobia, acquired intimacy deficiency syndrome (AIDS), heightened intimacy vulnerability (HIV), always-are-the-rightest, princess-itus, prince-itus, cystic me-and-mine-osis. Pretty soon we will be taking callers who have heard of more sexually transmitted relationship issues. After that, we'll talk about what a relationship and creationship are really all about."

I'm going to talk now about sexually transmitted relationship issues (STRIs). Just in case you've been living under a boulder, STRIs are about the biggest thing going in our male-dominated sex-sells culture. Before we talk about STRIs, however, let me help paint a picture of what a relationship is and could be. Now, for thousands of years people have tried to figure this out, and there are many definitions out there for you, so I'm going to describe relationships as zenfully as I can, as though I'm describing them to an alien. I hope I do a good job. If there are any aliens out there listening to the *Revival of The Fittest Radio Hour,* please call in or contact us through Twitter or Facebook. Let me take a deep breath. Okay, I'll tell you what it is. A relationship is one made two. If you have ever seen or know something about human beings coming together in the struggle to become one, you know something about a relationship. What makes relationships interesting are the new and ingenious ways that people can find to come together. Of course, what makes STRIs and relationships complex is that, after all, they involve two different humans. When relationships reach an inspired level, at times the two unite as one to produce a third little human being, so two become three. To reach such an inspired level is incredible.

It is hoped that the parents will teach their children about life, offer them every language they can, every area of study or science, every musical instrument, every sport, and every art and allow the children to select what they would like to learn. Those are wise parents. It is also hoped that the parents recognize their own shortcomings and work on them in order to become ideal and model adults for their children to follow. We can all hope for the best, for better tomorrows, even if we are presently stuck with a less-than-ideal situation—and most of us are. That is why, for many people, the journey of the first relationship is the start of the adventure into life. I once read a beautiful story about a young man who'd fallen in love. He walked to a river to take a look into the water and see his face, and for the first time he understood that there was something very different about his face that he couldn't quite explain. He had become self aware. It's a beautiful story. We all have a primary need to be loved and to love in return, and the people in a relationship have incredible roles and responsibilities to each other. Why? Because this person to whom you open your heart and expose your soul not only represents the inequity of love from your parents, but also the unfulfilled balance of every person in your life. Your boyfriend or girlfriend is your father, mother, brother, sister, uncle, grandfather, grandmother, boss, servant, enemy, and best friend, all rolled into one person. That's pretty poetic, especially when relationships and love allow us to see another side, an undeveloped side, an immature side of ourselves. We all have a foolish side. We all have an insecure side. We all have a temperamental side. That excelsior, tantalizing feeling we call "love" is so potent that it allows us to wear all of our masks and engage in all the aspects of our personalities at the same time. You only need one person to share that with. That is how powerful lovers are together, and that is how powerful love is when you compare it with who we often think we are.

The person you allow into your life also becomes all of your enemies, *all* of the people in your life who have tormented your consciousness only because you don't know how to forgive them. When you forgive people, you take back your energy of hate, blame, dependence, and fear and you finally become free of them. I'm not talking about "religious forgiveness," I'm talking about settling your debts and healing yourself. Personally, I can say that I've tried to forgive many people in my life, not because I want them to slap my other cheek and fall in love with them. That sounds a little like narcissism. I forgave them and learned to love them so that I could finally be free of them and take back my energy and my power, and it worked for me. Most of the time, when I talk about forgiveness, it goes over people's heads. It does have a religious dogmatic connotation, but let me tell you, there is no greater healing medicine than a heart that forgives. So if any soul out there in the world has come to represent every major relationship you've ever had, boiled down into one person, an ex-boyfriend or ex-girlfriend, I'd say you would be outstanding and incredibly wise to start forgiving them right this minute.

According to the Chinese, disease and death begin in the colon. The colon is analogous to the second seal or second chakra. So if you're into esoteric science, you could reason that disease begins in the attitudes formed in your second chakra. That is, disease manifests in the body when you give away your power of sensual pleasure and experience to another. Have you ever been in a relationship and desperately wanted your partner to pay attention to you because you were sick? Those kinds of attitudes contribute to disease and, dare I say, form the basis of disease itself. You are giving away your body by giving the authority and control of your sensual experience to another person. You are thus becoming *more* dependent. That is the second chakra on a really bad day, and we've all been there. I've written about relationships in my book *Slowness Gives Wholeness,* and we'll talk about that a little later.

This is advice for how to heal your body. A survey was once conducted on a large percentage of the world's population, endeavoring to figure out the number-one quality people look for in a relationship. Kindness was the most popular answer. So what brings us into a sexually transmitted relationship issue? Many, many things. Usually it's a lack of chemistry or common understanding. The people are trying to revive or live their first relationship with different people again and again and again, because they've never forgiven them. It is insecurity or deep-seated fear, jealousy, obsession, sexual obsession, manipulativeness, or codependence—root causes that destroy each and every failing relationship. A wise man I once knew said it best: "You are trying to possess another into possessing you." At the end of the day, the pure energy of this inferno dominates a love, relationship, or failing marriage, and that's when it's over. So how do we screen for STRIs? I'm going to help you with that. Find a pen and write these words down: vulnerophobia, acquired intimacy deficiency syndrome (AIDS), heightened intimacy vulnerability (HIV), always-are-the-rightest, princess-itus, prince-itus, cystic me-and-mine-osis. Pretty soon we will be taking callers who have heard of more sexually transmitted relationship issues. After that, we'll talk about what a relationship and creationship are really all about.

We have discussed the root causes of breakups and disease—possessiveness, jealousy, insecurity, fear, and all that. We've also looked into how the colon, vis à vis the second chakra, forms the basis of disease through disempowering attitudes. Now we'll look at the root causes of STRIs. Sensual experience becomes the basis of a relationship and causes you to 1) seek only sex; 2) use sex to improve self-esteem; and 3) use sex for leverage and survival. Let me say that I don't have anything against people who use sex for survival—not at all. If it works for you, and you and your partner are content and happy, all right! However, if you're at risk for sexual obsession and using sex for self-esteem and survival, you are at risk of an STRI. You're also probably not experiencing the more profound and deep healing and intimacy that major passion and undeniably wonderful sex offers. In other words, you might be cheating yourself, and that's just what these STRIs do. They help destroy relationships and, likewise, prevent you from building them.

Finding that your emotional energy has been in the wrong place is very unnerving and impedes the flow. Yet when you find your energy unobsessed, secure, and joyfully generous, then we're talking about the birth of a true lover and the kind of sex or intimacy that could end poverty, war, disease, depression—you know, save the world. How do these root causes manifest? Let's start with "always-are-the-rightest," one that I particularly struggle with from time to time. This is when open-mindedness flies out the window, and you are unable to listen or change. Then we look at HIV and AIDS—heightened intimacy vulnerability and acquired intimacy deficiency syndrome. What are they? HIV is an immensely powerful fear of being vulnerable that, in men especially, I find is related to the fear of death. AIDS is a progression of this fear and causes both men and women to become numb in a potentially intimate situation. You may not have ever experienced it, but let me assure you, it is really, *really* frustrating. If you're a man who has had AIDS, feel free to call in and discuss what it's like. The conditions are closely related to the syndrome called "vulnerophobia."

Vulnerophobia is when you have an aversion to intimacy, but you believe that you don't. Why? Probably because you have acknowledged yourself worthy in sports, money, social status, or sexual prowess. Now let's examine the word *vulnerability*. It means "susceptible to injury." A person with vulnerophobia might think he or she is safe, but sometimes one's preferred methodology of intimacy serves to protect and hide real vulnerability. We often find this in people who are deeply rooted in certain rituals. Perhaps in the beginning the ritual worked to resolve an emotional injury, but after enough repetition, the flavor's gone and it is simply that—repetition. Sex itself is an excellent example. Often a kiss on the lips is much more profound, personal, and intimate than sex that has become sort of repetitive. Finally, we have prince-itus and princess-itus. You may think these apply only to those with entitlement issues, but you'd be shocked to know that the other partner is, consciously or not, making him- or herself unavailable to receive.

That covers the relationship. Now, what is a creationship? Not too long ago I published a short story called *Union*. The story is about a man and woman in a tribe who agree to be married. They are sent into the forest with the barest provisions: knife, water, map, torch, and blanket. To have their marriage approved by the tribe, they have to survive in the deep jungle together for at least fifty days. They go on a thrilling adventure and end up married, and for the rest of their marriage they never once argue or fight. Au contraire—they were at peace. I was inspired to create *Union* by a reality show called *Pioneers* (anyway, I believe that was the name). In this reality show, a group of wealth-born people are charged with reenacting a journey up the Oregon Trail. They had no electricity, convenience items, or phones. During the show they made the very difficult journey together and even built a home together. They became so close through all of the challenges that many of them chose to sleep in the same rooms together. For the most part, they stopped arguing and began to show what could only be called "compassion." I thought it was a beautiful thing. If sand gets into your oyster, then with enough commitment, love, and spiritual surrender, you will find a shining pearl inside before the year is out. That's what a creationship is all about: *embracing challenges* and moving on the same pathway of personal growth. A creationship takes the sand—STRIs—throws it into an oyster called a relationship, coats the sand with the friction of wisdom and forgiveness, and produces the pearl. A creationship is the greatest form and only sustainable kind of relationship. If you are engaged in a legitimate creationship, we'd like you to call in and talk. Creationships are dynamic, very slow or very fast; they can have fewer colon problems; they can be sexual or nonsexual. They can produce gifted, brilliant children. They can set you on a course for evolution at light speed, and they can help expand your individual definition of unconditional love.

Now a creationship is a healthy relationship, and it actually promotes great health, but if you're in a good relationship and you want it to be *great*, you need good health. Thus you need a good relationship with *yourself*. When you heed Nature pyramid and strive for better sleep, nutrition, physical fitness, excellent hydration, and better breathing, you're vitally strengthening your connection to nature. What does vitality allow you to do? It gives you a chance to see beyond your discomfort level. Let's say an alcoholic meets a sober lady, and she brings him deeper sleep and some peace in his soul. This can help an alcoholic grow. Even if you're single or in a breakup, start taking better care of yourself and heal your relationship with your body and mind. You can get there through diet, exercise, hydrating, five rhythms dancing, or retreats, and you can find those golden moments when you know you're in a relationship with yourself and it is going beautifully.

Instead of drinking your sorrows with clear liquor, how would it feel if you took a short green juice cleanse? Instead of anticipating sleepless nights, laying awake in your bed, hearing sounds like someone's calling your name, it might be wiser to wear earplugs and a blindfold and go inside to spend some time with your heart. Hold it, soothe it, and feel and hear what it has to say. The voices in our head are so often triggered by sensory experience; a relaxed period of total sensory deprivation is excellent for calming the nervous system. You might have the best integrity in a relationship, and have a great relationship, but if health is your challenge and you are not embracing that challenge, you have left the creationship completely. One person who is growing cannot be in a creationship with another who is not. That is just a relationship, where the struggle is just to relate and not to create. It's not that you are from Venus and he is a Martian; you're just not creating with each other. That's the dilemma. It's also probably not as exciting as it used to be.

Now, before we take some calls, there is one more thing I want to talk about: breakups.

They're never easy. Sometimes they can be the best part or beginning of a real relationship, even if it's with yourself. Think about Henry VIII. For those of you who don't know his story, he cut the heads off his previous wives, because according to the Catholic Church, he could not divorce. Then he met a woman who changed his mind, a woman who, after breaking up with him, inspired him to talk with the Pope. Then he deviated from the Catholic Church and quite literally started his own religion just so he could divorce his current wife. Let's put that into context. When was the last time anyone created anything special to help them *break up* with someone, let alone a *religion?* What if this happened to you, and instead of cutting your girlfriend's or boyfriend's head off, you created "Johnathonism" or "Rebeccaism"? My point is, when you are in a dance with someone, you are investing in a belief system. Whether it is true belief or not, it's still a belief system into which you are putting your energy. Ending a relationship is like retracting your investment in it, and that's how it works. The best advice I could give you is, when you meet someone, and your lips and eyebrows float upward and you get bothered and hot, start out by asking them questions such as, "What do you want from me?" Then do them a favor and tell them what you want from them.

If you're serious, and you're serious enough about *being* serious, and you're looking for someone for a compatible creationship, just ask "What do you *need* from me?" and "What do I *need* from you?"

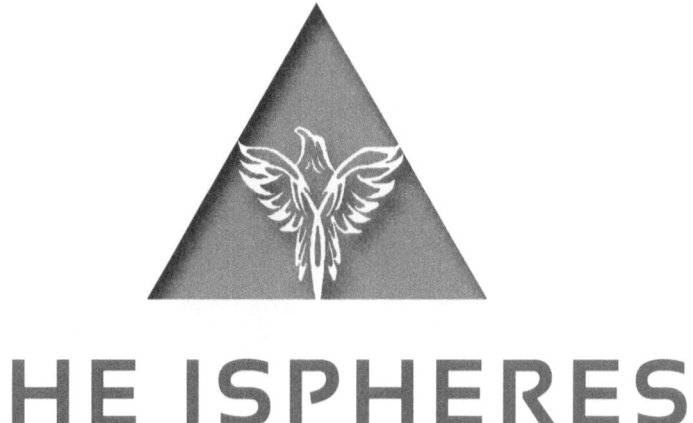

THE ISPHERES

"Quite naturally the young ladies were far more prepared than the gentlemen, who were in the habit of studying reclined, listening to music on their headphones, a beer in one hand, their feet up, a blunt in the other hand, the television on, wearing their shades, and reading the seventh edition Manual for Volatile Plutonium Extraction Upon Moon Landing.*"*

Unusual as it may seem, there are cultures in the Middle East that believe the best time for a man to impregnate a woman and acquire the responsibilities of fatherhood is at the ages of fifty, sixty, and seventy. Why? Perhaps they feel that at that point in their lives, they are wise enough to handle them. In India, the period of time that is considered "old age" is the most appropriate time to seek union with the divine. It is called the "age of walking through the forest." In the life cycle of trees, leaves fall from the lower and middle portions while the uppermost leaves huddle together in their final experience of heavenly light. I often wonder if that is similar to the experience of living as a wise old man. Do they all begin to reach for the stars? I ask myself.

This gentleness of old age, this spiritual thing, now seems to be under attack, not only by a dangerously unstable medical system but also by negligence. The West is socially conditioned to revere only what is "beautiful" and young. The astronauts of yesterday are fast becoming today's medicated and abandoned elders. So today I have a story to tell you.

The shuttle was called Fantastic Discovery. To ride it you had to be on your best of toes. Fantastic Discovery was the first under-18 space flight to the moon. Its passengers were a motley crew of princes, princesses, soldiers, joculars, sci-fis, rockers, and computer types. Their mission was to extract an unstable cache of plutonium from a crashed satellite that had landed somewhere on the dark side of the moon before it exploded. It was a race against the clock and against the Chinese who had been building their own under-18 shuttle, the U18 Discovery Ming, and the Russians and their U18 Discovery Shto. The bright minds given this job had been trained for this dangerous space rescue race online; all of them had taken several hours of home study courses on their Smartphones, iPads, laptops, peas, and pods. Quite naturally the young ladies were far more prepared than the gentlemen, who were in the habit of studying reclined, listening to music on their headphones, a beer in one hand, their feet up, a blunt in the other hand, the television on, wearing their shades, and reading the seventh edition *Manual for Volatile Plutonium Extraction upon Moon Landing.*

As you can imagine, most of the boys were sitting in the rear of the spacecraft. In truth, many had barely passed the physical examination. The ladies were better off, but nonetheless unfamiliar with riding in the cockpit, so this particular group of young lords and ladies had brought with them a dazzling array of personal electronic devices—Twitters, Googles, Nextels, iPhones, jPhones, kPhones, and the lot—and every one of them were texting each other, even as they sat right across from each other. My God. It was only a matter of time before the big clock started its ticking tock on the wall, and they opened the doors and let these confused teenagers enter the spacecraft. There they went, into the craft. Not a problem, not a problem at all!

They strapped themselves into the seats and turned off their electronic devices for the miraculous lifesaving ascent of the space shuttle Fantastic Discovery. Why, you ask? Because it is common knowledge that radiation from such electronic devices interferes with the instruments at the REGAL of the plane—I mean, space shuttle. I'll tell you this: not one of them could accept the possibility that their little electronic devices could ever permanently shut down for the remainder of their journey to the dark side of the moon.

[Sound effect of a shaky plane]

They're off. It's a great space embrace! They're racing, ascending, climbing to the heavens and parting clouds. The ride is getting more shaky [More effect], and then all at once, it calms. The four-wheel drive takes over, and the ladies and gentlemen may now turn on their electronic devices. However, they are advised, "as we pass through the Twittersphere, there will be no more tweeting." Recognizable shock appears on the faces of the ladies. The bad news continues: "And once we are clear of the Twittersphere, we will have to pass through the Facebookian radiation belt." "Oh my God," one passenger said. Within fifteen bloody minutes, not one of them could contact the collective Facebook community. Why? The Facebookian radiation had put an end to that, you see.

"Buckle your seat belts as we approach the Instagramosphere," the voice commands. The shuttle Fantastic Discovery began to reach the upper portions of the atmosphere. Catastrophic status messages were quickly posted for the comrades back on Earth. Never realizing they would be disconnected, the lot was understandably afraid. (That of course, tends to remind one of the adage, "There's no school like the good ol' fashion school of experience, oh baby"). Cutting through the Instagramosphere, they made their way toward the last gaseous radioactive upper layer of Earth: the bloody iSphere.

Suddenly [gasp] there is no more radiation. As the ladies rode a straight course to the dark side of the moon, some of the boys happened to take a look at the big, blue, wonderful emerald world below. It was as if they had never met their own mother. The Earth below was so great in its luminosity and form, and then…and then…. One little boy unconsciously repeated Will Smith's quote from *Independence Day*, "I've been waiting my whole life for this," and rather sounded quite like him, I'd say.

The ship's voice sounds an alert: "DANGER! DANGER! DANGER! The space shuttle is dangerously close to an unknown object in space! Danger!"

It was as though time slowed down. One little girl in the cockpit, right at the helm, looked down to see a beautiful text message from her boyfriend, seated in the rear of the space shuttle Fantastic Discovery. "What's happening?" it read. Right at that moment, however, coming fast and out of nowhere, the Russian space shuttle Discovery Shto smashed into the right side of Fantastic Discovery, putting an end to the rescue mission and catapulting both shuttles back to Earth in one hundred million pieces.

I feel that family is very important for sustaining our connection to nature. In fact, I argued with myself once to allow family, or human connection, as the eighth fundamental in my holistic health pyramid. The seven fundamentals are sleep, breathing, hydration, attitude, exercise, nutrition, and a connection to nature. It's interesting to note that the longest-lived demographic group in America is the not the whites but the Hispanics and Latinos. Why do Hispanics live for so long? If you know Hispanic families well enough, then you know that they do not always send their elderly off to assisted living. Their tightly knit family structure allows them to share wholesome meals together and learn how to live and resolve conflicts with one another. The Bureau of Labor Statistics has shown that during recessions, Hispanic women are actually much less responsive to corporate advertising and make *more* money during recessions. If *you* are trying to learn how to age gracefully, perhaps the holistic health pyramid plus family can really do the trick. The elderly have so much to offer. What greater thing can you teach than how to take care of yourself and to live healthy and with strong optimism? Youth and seniority are great times to be alive, and it all begins with how well you treat your mind and body, so today we are going to talk about how we get distracted from that concept, radiation protection, and how we can get ourselves back on track.

THE NATURE
PYRAMID

"Welcome to your connection to nature." You ask her, "Am I healed?" She responds, "You could be healed, but you have to go down now. Here, friend, you're on borrowed time. You have learned a little from each of the levels of the pyramid, of course. I suggest now that you put them into practice in the outside world, where there are no reminders. The lessons will remain hidden inside your soul."

Imagine that you are wearing a blindfold at the beginning of a great race, standing at the foot of an ancient pyramid. You're waiting at the door, and suddenly a cracking whip sends you running through the shadowed gates at top speed. Why do you run at top speed into the mystic holistic health pyramid? Because you're twenty-five years younger. You're on a search for the Holy Grail to heal your body, and to do that you must discover the source of the wind you feel. The air pressure on the first level is tremendous. You move blindfolded toward the sound of the wind blowing, and when you find it, the draft picks you up and blows you to the second level.

Here you can smell the sweet perfumes of powdered herbs, flowers, and cheeses. It makes you drowsy. You're so tired your feet can hardly move. Your head is bouncing off your chest. You want to fall asleep, but wait! You must complete your healing mission! So you search for the source of the aroma, and at last you find it. It must be a stew of boiling water. After smelling it, you fall into a deep sleep, but not all is lost; the magical aroma has melted the cloth from your eyes. You dip a cup into the pot to get a drink of this delicious brew that you imagine to be the Holy Grail. It's warm and refreshing. You begin to go for more, but you notice a hole under the Grail. It's the size of your body. In a moment you dive in and swim through tunnels until you come out on the third level of the holistic health pyramid.

There you find millions of frogs. They're everywhere, and they are... mating! Alas, for them there is no water to lay their eggs. But you find a door. Oh yes, a door. Painted on that door is a great blue wave. You look at it, and after a moment you decide to slowly, carefully, open it. Wham! You're hit by the wall of water, and millions of tiny frog eggs and legs are flying all over the place, but you saved them! Indeed, you saved the frogs!

You go on through the doors up into the fourth level, passing under a metal sign that reads, "Know Thyself." You're in a room. It's a room full of mirrors. However, to your delight there's another beautiful person of the opposite sex standing near you as well. You go to shake the person's hand, but you hit a mirror instead. You're walking through a room full of mirrors, searching for this partner, but hitting only illusions. You become angry, but then you smell what seems to be a delicious soup. Prudently, you close your eyes again and follow the aroma, and it leads you to yet another flight of stairs. Up you go into the fifth level. To your surprise, everybody in the holistic health pyramid is hanging out there. *It is so crowded,* you think to yourself. They're all chowing down, so you sit down to eat as well, but after you eat you're still hungry. However, the menu here is two thousand pages long, so long you could never get through it, so you eat, and eat, and eat, and eat, and eat.

Finally, you realize no one is going to stop you and lead you out of this level. You trek up the great stairs to great sixth level of the holistic health pyramid, and find you have walked right into NYSC Fitness! People are playing basketball, swimming, lifting, and running on treadmills. Everything is right and firm, the music and televisions are playing and the phones are ringing. Suddenly you notice a sweet little child walking around. She looks lost, almost as though she can't find her daddy or mommy. You walk up to her, and she looks at you, stops crying, looks serious, and points at you, saying, "How innocently you are making your way through the sixth level of health, my dear, but how many days will you just sit on a treadmill watching television in this artificial palace of exercise? How long will you eat and eat, rice bowl after rice bowl. How many hours will you spend hiding your flaws and using all your energy just to maintain the comfortable status quo? Do you really know how to drink from the water of life? How many nights have you slept that beautiful, heavenly, peaceful sleep of health? Do you love yourself enough to run straight through the wind, breathing its long, invisible hairs? Come with me if you want to know what healing is on the seventh level of the mystical, holistical pyramid, my friend."

On your way up to the seventh level, you hear the sound of the shore and the breathtaking sight of white, sparkling sands. You've arrived on a beach. Everyone is swimming in the sea together, breathing the wind, picnicking, resting, and sporting under the soft moonlight. Your little friend says, "Welcome to your connection to nature." You ask her, "Am I healed?" She responds,

"You could be healed, but you have to go down now. Here, friend, you're on borrowed time. You have learned a little from each of the levels of the pyramid, of course. I suggest now that you put them into practice in the outside world, where there are no reminders. The lessons will remain hidden inside your soul. If you stay on this beautiful beach forever, you will live only on borrowed time. Is that clear? However, if you leave now, you will have the chance to learn what it means to maintain health anywhere, anyhow, and forever and ever."

You look at her eyes, stunned that a little girl would say such things. Then she says, "Don't you think this is really what it's about? Do you agree?" "Well, I do," you answer. Thus you are healed temporarily, and you now must begin your journey down the pyramid. The journey of ascent we called *healing*, but the real journey is coming down off the mountain. The quest of descent is called *health maintenance and disease prevention*. Isn't that what it's really about? On your journey back down you are breathing happily through the gymnasium, joyfully tossing cold water over your head and back after a long and satisfying ball game, ahhh. It clears your head and allows you to focus on shooting the next basket. You feel calm and wild. The ball goes in every time, like water rolling up the shore or fresh air through the nostrils. The game is over, and you go back to the fifth level. Before you eat, you stretch and say a little prayer over the food. You're much happier than before and not as hungry as you used to be. You take a quick shower and make your way downstairs to the fourth level. In the house of mirrors, you again instantly find that partner and the two of you shake hands. However, this time the other person isn't made of glass but has a living body and a kind heart. Together you make it through the mirrored halls, guiding each other and listening to an unusual hum, a new sound in the air.

You get to the stairs and find that it's a chorus of the frogs! By listening, you can hear them singing below. You walk downstairs guided by an audible impulse. There among the frogs you find the deepest pool. This pool, as you recall, you made yourself. From there you sink into the underwater tunnel and exit the stew pot on the second level. To your surprise, the pot has morphed into a Jacuzzi! You relax in the Jacuzzi awhile before you return to the ground floor. You remember what the little girl said to you: "Healing is the journey up, but coming down, the journey is maintaining your health." *They are two different things,* you say to yourself. A cool breeze blows through the dark labyrinth of the ground floor. Those mysterious and invisible lips that once blew those aggravating breezes have moistened and tranquilized. You walk out the doors that you once ran blindly through, calmer, more centered and in control, more patient, and wiser than ever before.

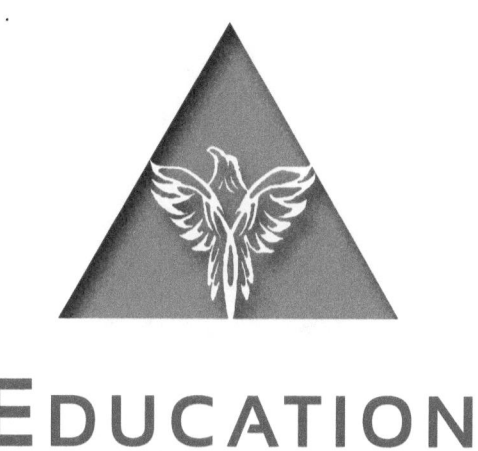

EDUCATION

"For better or worse, school is where the young become reflexive and subdued to authority. Our education system is cleverly designed as a miniature replica of the corporate world. We pass through promotions, or grades, when we earn their associated merits. Students compete for grades, ranking in class, high-stakes examination results, admission to honor societies, and entrance into institutions of higher learning. My philosophy is an option for the education system to transcend the pitfalls of competition altogether. With a strong emphasis on what matters most—health, mental acuity, informed decision making, and progressive learning techniques—the student body will naturally rise above its former competitive attitudes and radically improve the educational system itself within a few years."

Today I'm going to talk about the ways I think the education system in America could be improved.

Imagine you are in your junior year at Oxford University. You sit down to your lecture for the day, and the professor begins. About fifteen minutes later the professor stops and says, "Now I would like you to turn to the person on your left and discuss what you've learned thus far." The professor walks through his rows of students, and five minutes later says, "Now turn to the person on your right and do the same, and I'm listening."

After this he selects five students to the front of the class. He asks each of them to present what they have learned. Afterward, he tells the class, "Of these five students, how many of them are qualified to explain these concepts to a sophomore? How many of them are qualified to explain these concepts to a ninth-grade student? Fifth grade? What about a second-grade student?" The class makes its preferences clear, and only two of the five students could teach the material to a fifth grader or a second grader. Their names are put on a list, and the professor begins teaching again, only to repeat this same interactive learning process fifteen minutes later. What happens? The students who made the list do not have to teach sophomores, freshman, or second graders, and they receive good marks in class for the day. However, the students who have not shown a high aptitude for learning the material are put to task with teaching younger students. When the younger students are tested on the material learned, their grades will then affect the older students' teachers.

This kind of learning/teaching is called *interactive learning,* and it is in use at several universities around the world, such as Oxford University. It is highly effective because it forces immediate comprehension of the subject and ensures that students are paying attention. It also provides the teacher with a brief refrain. Interactive learning is modeled upon how the brain actually works. The human brain often does not distinguish between external and internal stimulation. In other words, when the brain learns, it is teaching itself. Can you imagine a school like this that both teaches and learns at the same time, at an accelerated rate? I love this little school, and it is the beginning of a revolution and evolution in the education system.

I think students deserve a more progressive curriculum that includes finances, logic, and current events. Most students go on to give away their own hard-earned money to someone else who will then supposedly build a retirement fund for them. This is one of many not-so-bright ideas coming from the corporate world, especially in light of these trying economic times. Students therefore should keep abreast on current events and come to these rational decisions on their own with regard to their future well-being. A rigorous course in logic can help to emphasize the need for deeper concentration and reasoning so the students can avoid injustices and flaws in the system and assess their own financial situations. A progressive curriculum could help students make informed decisions at a younger age and would tie in very well with interactive learning. Imagine a group of fourth graders having an informed conversation about the cost of living and what responsibilities they could pursue and realistically enjoy?

I believe yoga, nutrition, and the holistic health pyramid of breathing, sleeping, hydration, attitude, nutrition, fitness, and nature should be taught in every school system. If it can improve the employees of several Fortune 500 companies like Google, General Electric, and HBO, making them twice as productive, healthier, and far more creative, how great of a leap is it to bring it to school?[5] Then students could explain nature's values to other students in an interactive learning scenario. What if students were encouraged to take excellent care of their greatest asset: their brains? What if they were taught to avoid dietary excesses and encouraged toward hydration, omega threes from flaxseed, granular lecithin, and sulfur compounds from garlic leeks and onions—all nutrients that can do wonderful things for cognitive ability. In fact, there is a famous study that demonstrated that the more a person concentrates on a particular subject, the more phosphorous

---

[5] Walton, Alice. How Yoga May Save the US Trillions of Dollars. Available from: http://executiveyogainc.com/how-yoga-may-save-the-us-trillions-of-dollars/

is found in his or her urine. In other words, the phosphatidylcholine present in granular lecithin is sort of like brain fuel. Let's not forget about slow, deep breathing and a short routine of concentration exercises. Adding such exercises into students' curriculum would provide them with a risk-free option to improve the quality of their lives.

Jerry Seinfeld once said that "Grades are not the value of school experience. Mental exercise is." Nobody could have said it any better. We learn to cogitate in school and to complete tasks using mental faculties. I think this is where schools could benefit the most. We test our students on the basis of knowledge. Why not test them on the basis of cognitive ability as well? Let's have required memory and attention span tests. In order to avoid self-judgment, students should take cognitive tests twice weekly, keeping their results personal. This would help them tremendously because it would allow them to see that the capability of the mind is not so set in stone and that it can be improved and built upon. It is not predetermined. The students may learn to equate mental exercise with training for sports, and perhaps a standardized routine of mental exercises will improve athletic performance as well.

What would be greater than students who understand their minds, gauge their abilities, and willfully improve themselves without so much emphasis on competition and the rigors of conforming to public opinion? Concentration is really the keynote of all mental ability. From rehabilitation, increasing worker productivity and improving students without also improving focus, your results will be a failure. Attention-deficit disorder (ADD) is a particularly unnerving concept in the system that should be reevaluated immediately. ADD is unpredictable by the standards of psychology. It can't be tested in the classroom without six months of observation. However, focus exercises and attention span tests can be done in class. Ultimately, well-being in body and mind is everything. These are my suggestions: First, students should be exposed to a more progressive curriculum that includes finances, logic, and current events. Second, students should engage in interactive learning. Third, students should be introduced to the value of mind-body activities. Fourth, students should be periodically tested with regard to cognitive ability.

For better or worse, school is where the young become reflexive and subdued to authority. Our education system is cleverly designed as a miniature replica of the corporate world. We pass through promotions, or grades, when we earn their associated merits. Students compete for grades, ranking in class, high-stakes examination results, admission to honor societies, and entrance into institutions of higher learning. My philosophy is an option for the education system to transcend the pitfalls of competition altogether. With a strong emphasis on what matters most—health, mental acuity, informed decision making, and progressive learning techniques—the student body will naturally rise above its former competitive attitudes and radically improve the educational system itself within a few years. These techniques are in practice some places around the world and gaining a substantial reputation. By loosening and perhaps removing the shackles of competition, students would flourish within their own lives.

If you really think about it, right now young children in the Amazon jungle are whittling to make their own wooden toys to play with while our fourth graders are busy filling in the colors and writing the same damned sentence over and over again. I don't have all the answers, and I'm not suggesting that I do. What I do have is a personal insight, and I'd like to find out what you think as well. Even if you call in to challenge me, do so, because that's also important for learning also.

Today it seems that if you can stand before a class with a couple of notes handy and a long list of simple facts, you will make a great teacher. Memorization, enumeration, and high-stakes examination are overvalued, and experience, participation, teamwork, and spontaneous creativity are really lacking emphasis. Yet experience is really the best teacher. If we do nothing really innovative or original to revive the education system in America, everything will topple. Many research studies have shown that the American education system is producing mediocre students when compared with the rest of the civilized world. There are more frightening statistics that also speak to this fundamental problem. These statistics are fully referenced in my book *Self Determination*. Six out of ten college students use drugs. One out of every four Americans is said to be suffering from a mental illness, which equates to almost fifty-eight million Americans. One in every seventeen people is said to have a serious mental illness. Twenty million women and ten million men suffer from a significant eating disorder sometime in their lives. In the past two decades, virtually all mental health statistics have been on the rise. From 1999 to 2010, the middle-aged suicide rate increased a dramatic 30 percent. A June 2013 Gallup poll revealed that 70 percent of Americans hate their jobs or have "checked out" of them.

What are the problems in the education system, according to the experts? They are bullying, failing students, standardized testing, poor teacher salaries, and poor budgeting. These can be solved with some insight and ingenuity emphasizing informed decisions, health, mental acuity, and interactive learning over typical distractions, lack of student desire, and flaws in the system. These things are what got us into this mess. Distractions like cell phones, drugs, and television have been proven to affect one's health and lead to eating unhealthy foods and sometimes severe weight gain. If a high school student is in the habit of studying reclined, listening to music on the headphones, a beer in one hand, feet up, a blunt in the other hand, the television on, wearing shades, and reading *Apology* by Plato, that student is in desperate need of health, mental acuity, informed decisions, and interactive learning. Third graders could tell you that—if you taught them properly, that is.

I would love to see students creating folk remedies, sea salt, vinegar, hydrogen peroxide, even olive oil. Perhaps there are a few future healers, scientists, or chefs in that class. Now we're talking about learning from experience. Personally, I would love to see a school of students interactively learning about our environment, poverty, war, leadership qualities, and environmental awareness. I would love to see the fourth grade teach the third, and the third grade teach the second, and so on. Jean Rousseau, a philosopher, once said that we learn from three things: men, things (or experience), and nature. If in school we learned to protect and accelerate our own natures, we accelerate our learning through experience, and thus accelerate our learning from men. There are no limits. I would love to see students creating everyday household items in school.

I believe every student by the beginning of the sixth grade should write their own autobiography in ten thousand words. This is equivalent to two months of weekly essays. I believe yoga, nutrition, and the holistic health pyramid should be taught in every school system, at home, and in every classroom. If it can improve the employees of a Fortune 500 company, it can also help our struggling students. Think about it. It's time for new ideas that run contrary to the status quo. That's why we are here at Revival and that's also why it is so important to educate the youth.

AN ENVIRONMENTALLY SAFE HUMAN

"Why has there been an over six hundred percent increase in reported autism cases in the United States just in the past twenty years? One in eighty-eight children now is diagnosed with autism spectrum disorder. Exactly why have attention-deficit/hyperactivity disorder, autism, dyslexia, and mental retardation reached epidemic proportions? In July 2010, the Centers for Disease Control and Prevention determined that the average American has 212 synthetic chemicals coursing through his or her blood or urine—seventy-five of which had never before been measured for toxicity. The other 137 synthetic chemicals are linked to increases in prostate and breast cancers, diabetes, heart disease, lowered sperm counts, the early onset of puberty, and other common diseases and disorders. How many more hundreds of synthetic chemicals do we need to find in the umbilical cord of the average baby before society takes action?"

As much as a personal connection to nature can help you lose weight, beautify the body, improve athletic performance, increase productivity, enhance the imagination, enhance the thinking mind, and save the environment, there's a benefit to my holistic health pyramid that exceeds all of these beautiful qualities. You are probably thinking it's peace of mind, but not really. The greatest benefit in the health pyramid, far greater than any other, is that it allows you to keep your body environmentally safe. Why? Why is an environmentally safe body the most fundamental gift from nature? Without a safe, secure body, you could end up a strong and beautiful corpse, a little before your time, with an excellent reputation. You could die without living in an environmentally safe body.

So let's try to understand this wonderful thing called "the connection to nature." As you know, it's the main theme of our show. There are seven fundamentals for health that result in a connection to nature: breathing, sleeping, drinking, attitude, eating, fitness, and healthy sensory stimulation. Healthy sensory stimulation could include hygiene, sunlight, clean water, grounding, or physical comfort. If you can help yourself enough to really learn what a connection to nature is about, you can unplug yourself from your distractions and addictions and focus on what really matters most. Without a deep awareness of the seven fundamentals and their crown prince, the connection to nature, we are nice, complacent, and predictable cogs in a wheel building up some fortune for some gentlemen in Abu Dhabi while we buy and sell stocks and Halloween candy. We can all do better for ourselves by looking at how well we eat, workout, sleep, hydrate, deal, and breathe, no question about it. If you know that you have made some mistakes in the past with your health, that is why we are here at the Revival Hour, and thank you very much for listening. I wonder; if an environmentally safe body was a top priority for every individual, would the world suddenly and unexpectedly transform overnight? Absolutely. In fact, if 70 percent of the people in the world only attempted to clean up part of their act, we'd live in a brave new world. Why? That 70 percent would set an example for the remaining 30 percent. Today it is very much the opposite in the US of A, where people are watching television an average of six hours a day and are not the least bit curious about strengthening their connection to nature. Today it is the 1 percent that is setting an example for all. There is nothing wrong with trying to be financially successful and well respected, but compared with having an environmentally safe body, that's nothing.

Most of us live in a toxic world. It's the truth. The US government has banned only ten ingredients for cosmetics, whereas Europe has outlawed 1,372! More startling, the United States actually allows the cosmetics manufacturers to test their products themselves to be sure they are responsible for following Food and Drug Administration (FDA) guidelines. Also, the European Union has banned certain antibacterial soaps that contain triclosan, but the FDA has yet to take a firm position on the subject. The FDA takes years to reach such conclusions. Keep in mind that triclosan is also found in mouthwash, toothpaste, and toys. Today, to remove triclosan products from the market would compromise a billion-dollar industry. In spite of this, most of the soaps, shampoos, household cleaning products, laundry detergents, synthetic fabrics, cosmetics, flame retardants, x-ray machines, toothpastes, deodorants, and fuel exhaust that contain known pollutants are not addictive and are not primary causes for our interior environmental pollution. So what is? The top culprits here are sugar, television, and radiation. Overwhelming evidence shows that sugar and radiation from electric screens are both, in fact, addictive. Furthermore, each of these toxic entities delays or lessens the effect of deep, natural rest and restoration.

Why has there been an over six hundred percent increase in reported autism cases in the United States just in the past twenty years? One in eighty-eight children now is diagnosed with autism spectrum disorder. Exactly why have attention-deficit/hyperactivity disorder, autism, dyslexia, and mental retardation reached epidemic proportions? In July 2010, the Centers for Disease Control and Prevention determined that the average American has 212 synthetic chemicals coursing through his or her blood or urine—seventy-five of which had never before been measured for toxicity. The other 137 synthetic chemicals are linked to increases in prostate and breast cancers, diabetes, heart disease, lowered sperm counts, the early onset of puberty, and other common diseases and disorders. How many more hundreds of synthetic chemicals do we need to find in the umbilical cord of the average baby before society takes action? In 2007, suicide became the third leading cause of death for young people ages fifteen to twenty-four. What has caused this dramatic increase? When do we decide to test our tap water for drugs, noxious chemicals, parasites, or heavy metals? According to George Washington University's Face the Facts Initiative, 850 billion gallons of wastewater enter our public water supply every year. By the way, that is 13.6 trillion glasses, which brings us to roughly forty-five thousand glasses per American per year. The US Environmental Protection Agency (EPA) has publicly stated that our water treatment facilities will require $500 billion in maintenance and new capital investment by 2020. Keep in mind that in the past twelve years we have doubled our defense spending in America. Be aware that public water supplies in forty-two US states are contaminated with 141 unregulated chemicals for which the EPA has never established safety standards. Why do Americans make up an estimated 5 percent of the world's population yet produce an estimated 30 percent of the world's waste while using 25 percent of the world's resources? Why do conventional sources of media not report on any of this?

It's obvious we are living in a world of limited resources where life, liberty, and the pursuit of happiness are determined by a struggling majority. Ask yourself: if life, liberty, and the pursuit of happiness come at the expense of health, what food are happiness, liberty, and life? If an environmentally safe body were sacrificed on the altar of the so-called American dream, who would want to dance under fireworks on the fourth of July? The old American icon James Dean once said, "Live as if you were to die tomorrow." Here's the problem with that statement. What if you were *not* going to die tomorrow? What if instead you were going to die in fifty years? How about that for nature's self-deterministic propaganda? Live like you're going to die in sixty years. How about, "Live as if you were to wake up tomorrow" or "Live as if you were to never die." We can create a poster or a T-shirt that says, "I will live eternally from now on." I can see t-shirts printing all the way from here. I think many people, unfortunately, are so uncomfortable with their station in life, and thus so disconnected from nature, that they unconsciously feel as if they will die tomorrow. That, my friends, is no way to live at all. A few months ago I wrote a story about a world where everyone worshipped homeless people. Isn't that what life would be like if we lived as if we were to die tomorrow? We would have life in the kingdom of bums. Yet the unfree world worships wandering pacifists like Jesus, Buddha, and Moses. Just some food for thought.

It would be true liberty for the soul if you told yourself tonight, "No I'm not going to die tomorrow. I'm not going to die for at least thirty-five years. Forget dying tomorrow." When you've had enough of this self-destructive propaganda about dying tomorrow, you can start to build into your future, save your energy, plan ahead, and do the smart thing and strengthen your connection to nature. Perhaps you could sit for an hour each day and silently meditate for the simple truth of nature to expose itself. If you started today, in three years life still might not be without challenges. However, if you honor yourself long enough, your life will have aged beautifully like sweet wine

It starts with an environmentally safe body. The only way to really pull this off is by observing the seven fundamentals (breathing, sleeping hydration, attitude, nutrition, exercise, and a connection to nature). If you do pull it off, who cares about the American dream? You can care about *your* dream, because that's more important. Nature is your guardian, your nurturer, the one who gave you life. A connection to nature improves the soul and is the ambition of the soul. So if you're ready and you've decided to live for your soul, rather than the whole, we can start figuring out how to make this machine work properly.

The first three fundamentals are air quality, rest quality, and water quality. Air quality on Earth is a very large dilemma. Before you do anything else, purchase some indoor plants for where you rest. Peace lilies and snake plants are my favorite. I usually recommend seven plants per person, which is about enough to live inside a bubble with them and survive. Austin Air and IQ Air are excellent brands of air filters, and I recommend them as well. Once you have those plant vibrations in your room, you will find yourself more relaxed and have an easier night's sleep. If you include melatonin, GABA, B vitamins, L-tyrosine, L-tryptophan, ear plugs, and a sleeping mask that also covers your ears, it really doesn't matter what kind of mattress you have, rest assured. You should also think about stretching a little before you sleep, and make sure that you wind your nights down, turn off the big screens and sounds, do not eat or eat lightly, turn the lights down, walk slow, think slow, and turn the phone off if you can. It doesn't matter how well you think you sleep, the older we get the less natural melatonin hormone we produce, so any assistance will bring you magnificent results. This is how you keep the body environmentally safe for fundamentals one and two. Avoid sugar, stimulants, and eating large meals at night. Why? Because these are all things that prevent the body from properly restoring itself and enjoying its eight hours of slow, deep, fully unconscious breathing.

When it comes to water quality, there are enough challenges on Earth to be aware of. Many people ask me what kind of filtration they should get. In every circumstance, quantity is more important than quality. A shower filter, ceramic filter, a cheap distiller, and a homemade sand-activated charcoal filter tend to go a very long way and are much more reliable than a four-thousand-dollar machine that claims to do it all. That is not to say that a four-thousand-dollar ionizer isn't an incredible investment in one's health, because it certainly is, but we want to cover all the bases in this world, and we want that pure H_2O to make it through the toughest holes and cracks in your metaphorical desert. I regularly shower with filtered water. When I don't, my skin is dry. The food I cook with filtered water tends to taste better. My dog, when given a bowl of filtered water and a bowl of tap water, will always drink the filtered water first. So the third fundamental for an environmentally safe body is to get yourself good, clean, and refreshing water.

Now we arrive at attitude, the "wild card" fundamental I like to call it. In an aspirational pyramid, attitude would be number one, because wouldn't we all like to smile and live forever healed? Most people, however, are not strong enough in their focus to actually make that happen. They must rely on the body's metabolism. In other words, people won't be smiling if they miss two days of sleep and water—most of us, at least. Really, disease comes from a dis-easement. It's a misappropriation of energy. A simple lie detector may show how much your mind and attitude transform your body. Disease is *dis*-ease. Yes, that is a common phrase I like to use these days, but there are other ways to make that connection. You could say if you feel ineffective, you might be infected. If you find a pathology, study the path from whence it came, baby. These are just other ways of saying what the sages have always said: Your thoughts matter. Consciousness and energy create the nature of reality. You may work out, meditate, practice qi gong or tai chi, or listen to music. It's always better to renew your spirit than to keep visiting the same people and places that hide it from you.

This leads us to the fifth most important fundamental: what you eat. I say it is the fifth fundamental because it is, although many would say it's the first, because the wholesome and nutritive quality of the standard American diet does not really exist. If you walk into any supermarket, 85 percent of everything contains wheat or sugar. Anyone can figure out that if you eat too much sugar you disrupt the balance of energy in your body, because oxygen and sugar create energy. That's why people who eat too much sugar experience a sugar rush and then pass out. All of these foods are called comfort foods, and yet they do not satisfy the craving that your body really has. Think of your Thanksgiving dinner. Would you eat a plate of turkey, potatoes, collard greens, yams, and fresh corn, or would you eat pie? If you chose dinner over pie, you were in touch with your natural appetite mechanism in that moment. If you were to go on a short detox, or cleanse, you could help improve that natural taste mechanism inside your body. Then you might start to crave nature's number one elixir of environmental security: chlorophyll. The more chlorophyll you consume in your diet, the more resilient you are to the effects of air pollution, radiation, and general toxicity. It's a three-in-one knockout elixir. I prefer wheat grass juice, powdered kelp, dandelion leaf, nettles, and alfalfa more than any other supplement. I typically recommend four ounces of wheatgrass per day if you can stomach it. If you can get enough raw, nutritious foods that contain enough chlorophyll or other photo nutrients, you will improve your natural appetite and won't be constantly craving other foods with scant mineral content. Recently I came up with a fantastic and simple, natural crave-blocking powder. All you have to do is combine equal parts spirulina or any of my chlorophyll suggestions with Ceylon cinnamon, beet root, and stevia powder. Make sure they are as fresh as possible.

It always feels good to be satisfied after a meal, you know? Soups are also a great way to handle cravings, and so is apple cider vinegar, or lemon turmeric and bee pollen in hot boiled water, or saffron herb. In my book *Folk Remedies for the Modern Age* I created the chlorophyll pollen fast for people who struggle with food cravings, and it's worth picking up and reading it if you struggle with them as well.

Fundamental number six is exercise. If exercise came in a pill, it would be the most popular health supplement in the world. Recently *60 Minutes* did a short on high-intensity, short-duration exercise. It shows that people who sprint, swim, cycle, or even dance at very fast, very vigorous speeds, top speeds, are getting some remarkable, incredible, outstanding health benefits. If you are able to do it, it is worth getting on a cycle to give it a try. My favorite forms of exercise are five rhythms dancing, Bikram yoga, basketball, and beach soccer. We'll talk about what five rhythms dancing is later in the show.

You might know that beekeepers are the longest-lived professionals in the world. It is absolutely true. What better way to define connection to nature? Did you know that bees are genetically programmed to overproduce because they have adapted to predators eating their pollen propolis and honey. If there are not predators, bees will eventually overproduce and even die. You know, some animals trek for hundreds of miles just for honey. I think it is worth the trek of one hundred miles, if you are that distant, for a connection to nature. If you can keep your body environmentally safe and eat, drink, sleep, breathe, feel, workout, and enjoy nature, you can enjoy the fruits of your own labor.

No Defeat,
No Surrender

"Vision and I are purveyors, organizers, artists, and storytellers. We're here and in the zone. There's enough history and experience between the both of us to make this kind of quality program last, and I think it will. I think it will be an important program."

Every family of every major world leader, including the Obamas, the Romneys, and the Blairs, prefers unpolluted, fresh, natural, organic food and purified water. Be assured there is nobody in the White House drinking water from the tap. In fact, thanks to the handiwork of our beautiful and bright First Lady Michelle Obama, the White House roof now includes hanging gardens where tomatoes, lettuce, cucumbers, onions, and hundreds of other vegetables are grown. I might start to call it the "Green House," especially if Michelle Obama adds a few more fundamentals into the domestic life such as sleep quality, air quality, and inspirational activities. What are those inspirational activities I'm talking about? I'm glad you asked. Maybe she could start a library with some of the most inspirational autobiographies of all time, such as Nelson Mandela's autobiography *A Long Walk to Freedom,* Helen Keller's *The Story of My Life,* or biographies of Benjamin Franklin, Malcolm X, Martin Luther King, or even Miles Davis. Perhaps she could collect a few of the most inspiring films of all time, such as *It's a Wonderful Life, To Kill a Mockingbird, E.T., Breaking Away, Miracle on 34th Street, Amélie, Saving Private Ryan, The Bridge on the River Kwai, Gandhi,* or *Ray.* I can visualize the holistic health pyramid on the wall in the White

House for all to be reminded of their connection to nature. Nothing would make me happier.

Today we have 1.4 million veterans who are unemployed. New York City police officers are making much less than forty thousand dollars per year, and they have to buy their own uniforms, boots, night sticks, and guns. These are people who defend our lives! Living healthy sounds like quite a commodity for those who are just barely surviving. The problems, as bad as they are, can be compounded when weekends are spent running around drinking beer, sweating for bigger muscles, and watching someone eat fifty hot dogs in nine minutes. All of us are being conditioned to destroy ourselves, and it's really time we put an end to the game. Soon there will be nowhere to turn. After Hurricane Sandy devastated the northeastern United States in 2012, our government told us that rising ocean levels will bring on larger and more frequent storms. Climatologists are warning us of such a change. It seems that a shift is on its way. Increased incidences of earthquakes, hurricanes, volcanoes, famine, floods, and solar flares are leading to food shortages, hazardous-waste release, and epidemics all over the world. Are you informed? Are you prepared? You need to be.

On October 25, 2011, Betty Sutton, a member of the Ohio House of Representatives, told the US House of Representatives, "Every day in the United States, we are losing fifteen factories." The last economic recession saw a total loss of $72 trillion worldwide. Householders in the US alone lost $19.2 trillion, according to the US Treasury Department website. Moreover, new heat records were set in all fifty states. New drought records also were set in all fifty states. You might still be feeling the heat from the recession of 2011; however, money is not the only resource drying up at home. It is time to go beyond what is comfortable. When the people begin to lose it all, there will be no option for surrender or defeat. You see, it's a game, a game of how to hold a massive population just above the tipping point long enough to extract all the resources, energy, and admiration that they can. In other words, it's a terrible game of "How can we feed off of them?" There is an answer for people who understand manipulation, no matter how subtle it is. There's an option for people regardless of whether they come from the highest or lowest station in life. That option is a connection to nature. What does a connection to nature require? Knowledge and sovereignty. I'll explain.

The only reason people made the long journey over to America was for freedom. The people here yearned to live on with the good Earth and beholden to no one, no king, and no commodity. That's the spirit that rings in Whitman's words, the original United States with honest qualities of self-effacement, thrift, and originality. What happened? Now our president and our mayor are telling us to go out and shop for Christmas to boost the economy. It's sort of like telling a morbidly obese child to run and play in a candy shop. Sometimes you just can't afford it. That yearning for independence is still in our genes, and I'm not talking about these Levis. Rebuilding your life is not an overnight gig. As I like to say, its slowness which gives wholeness. Every day for the past few years, I've met with people who were struggling to survive and at the same time trying hard to discover what it means to be healthy and discover a much more profound connection to nature.

The road back home to nature is fraught with difficulty. My career, as I have made it, isn't about keeping one person ahead. It's about pulling everybody up. I've written about very common household things that you can use to improve your health and hygiene. I've written about the top seven preventable causes of death in America, and how you can prevent them. I've written about better sleep and fundamentally improving your health with simple, accessible advice and language—no designer goofs, no gimmicks, *no lies, no high prices,* nothing fairy written or airy written. I don't mince words. It is the people's house. It is the people's country. I'm not here to waste anybody's time, especially considering the extraordinarily short attention span of the average barely surviving American. I want everybody to win in this game, I truly do. When I see thousands from my generation on a downward spiral into complacency, lethargy, addiction, and depression, it just encourages me. When I see the homeless man walking by a river where thousands of fish literally swim through each day, it makes me sit down and wonder. Knowledge is power, and the more high-quality knowledge you get, the more sovereign and free you can become. High-quality knowledge: That's what this work here is about. Vision and I are purveyors, organizers, artists, and storytellers. We're here and in the zone. There's enough history and experience between the both of us to make this kind of quality program last, and I think it will. I think it will be an important program.

What is this high-quality knowledge I'm talking about? It's sort of like saying "feed a man a fish and he'll eat for a night; show a man how to fish and he'll eat for a lifetime." When it comes to health and wellness, many of us are not putting the right pieces into the puzzle. We are. There's no shortage of integrity here, we're all walking our talk. So are the people that we invite on the show. That's our commitment to you. You're going to get to see and hear about the breath of life and that mental health and attitude is everything. You know these fundamentals, attitude and breath, are instinctually related; there are many ways to breathe and only one way to pay attention, but the breathing is made better through concentration. Concentration is made stronger by the breathing. Breathing and focus are the heaven and Earth, yin and yang, the positive and negative of a life committed to strengthening your connection to nature. Take a breath—a deep one—a slow, deep breath and listen.

There are three great pillars of civilization: art, justice, and medicine. Our mission is to progress and fully embody those pillars, that great trisophany. With justice, you can avoid and defend yourself from crime and manipulation. With art, you can inspire. With medicine, you can heal. Think of this show as a gateway to the foundation, the basement floor, of the civilized world. That's art, justice, and medicine, and that's why they call it the underground. So get yourself comfortable and enjoy the ride.

PAIN

"Once a scientist and philosopher named Descartes took an afternoon to cut up a living dog in order to understand how the heart muscle functioned. Later on in history, Descartes would champion the "mechanistic view" of life, in which all creatures are essentially soulless and predetermined by biological motives. Today this is the orthodox perception."

When a wolf breaks its leg, it finds a cave to lie down in. The wolf will stay in the cave for weeks and fast on water if necessary. The wolf will wait this long or longer before taking a few careful steps through the dark cave, and then it will walk around inside the cave for days. Finally, when the leg is healed, the wolf will come out of the cave, strong on its leg. When a bird loses a hatchling to a predator, or lays a sterile egg, the bird will weep, and it will shake when it weeps. The same is true for a dog that has experienced physical trauma. The same weeping, shaking motions and learning are actually true for many advanced species of animals on Earth. In fact, when I look at beached whales and dolphins on the news, I find myself wondering what kind of pain they experienced that caused them to do away with themselves in large groups. It's troubling to say that fish of all sorts are beaching themselves. I had a theory about it; these creatures, these animals are not killing themselves just to make a statement. Perhaps they intuitively understand that humanity has destroyed the food chain and are actually trying to save the Earth by allowing the foundations of our food chain, plankton, algae, and small fish, to grow a little faster than they are being exterminated. When I watch them destroy themselves on heavily populated beaches, I understand that nature has an extraordinary intelligence as well as a dark sense of humor.

People, what have we to learn about pain? Lots, I'd say. A few months ago I was sitting in my psychology class at Montclair State University, and I raised my hand to the question, "How does stress work?" It seemed to me that I was going to share the simplest answer, one that wouldn't offend any other students, wouldn't shock them, or may even interest them. When I was called on, I said, "Stress can accumulate. You know, if you don't handle your stress when something like traffic, arguing, or extra work comes around, it doesn't magically disappear. It can come back stronger." Without expecting it, I looked around to see almost every student look down, swallow, and avoid my glance. What does the common person understand about stress or about pain? How does it accumulate? Can it transform? Can it influence your environment? Does it ever end? Why is pain incomprehensible to us and not to nature? I believe in the future. I work and hope for the best. I believe that in the future there will only be one form of psychology, and that form of psychology will understand exactly what pain is. Suffering and fear of suffering sit at the heart of all human problems. Today we can call ourselves experts if we know the source of that suffering and can identify its effect in our lives. You know the person who says, "I think I married my mother or father"? (That Freudian dilettante.) That person can understand pain to the point of identifying a pattern a majority of the time.

I wonder; if pain were a flower, how would it grow? Would it be wounded by an unkind word? How would it die? We really know nothing about pain. Some of the so-called brightest students at Stanford University were once experimenting and researching psychological motives and decided it would be a good idea to lock half the volunteers in a jail and have the other half work as guards. They told them to play it seriously, and then they watched what happened. The result was the infamous Stanford prison experiment where unnecessary pain and cruelty were inflicted by the student body upon itself in what could have been the most abstract research experiment. Then there are the Milford experiments that are available on YouTube. They are both mindblowers. Still, it makes me wonder: can anyone understand pain if they haven't hurt enough or been hurt enough? I think the answer is no, quite resoundingly. We can call it what it is. We can call it the shadow. If you take a brief look at history, you will see that human beings are perhaps the most emotionally disturbed creatures alive on Earth. From the beginning of civilization humanity has learned to harness from nature the means with which to eradicate hunger, poverty, and its associated challenges. Yet despite Ancient Egypt's impeccable model of agriculture, the body politic of Ancient Greece, and the recordkeeping of Sumer, the vast majority of our ancestors had to fight to survive without the benefit of knowledge, and they still do so today. It comes down to pain again, the state of inner suffering. The blues, if you will.

Why do people have panic attacks, throw nervous fits, or unexpectedly cry? Because they are without factor KOS: Knowledge Of Self. Why does terror strike in the middle of our dreams? Why do people feel abandoned, even when they are alone? Why do words create deep wounds that never heal, and why do people ignore the pain they feel? Today we want to describe the life cycle of inner suffering. It's a lot like peeling the layers of an onion. As you peel the onion away, we discover the nature of our sorrow, or fear, or pain. Most often we discover that the fundamental nature of our pain is really a common one: mortality, abuse of power, manipulation, loneliness, smallness, bigness, addiction, fear, and fear of the unknown. Whatever it is, we all have it to some degree or another. Just to realize that we all share the same seed of pain, if you respect and love yourself enough, can be *life changing*, terribly life changing.

Most of us don't get it, however, and there's a reason for that. Once, a scientist and philosopher named Descartes took an afternoon to cut up a living dog in order to understand how the heart muscle functioned. Later on in history, Descartes would champion the "mechanistic view" of life, in which all creatures are essentially soulless and predetermined by biological motives. Today, this is the orthodox perception, and it's hard to refute when we are controlled by the television, the clock, the boss, the government. If you're struggling to survive, you're not free. In spite of this obvious flaw in the system and the system's rhetoric, there is this wonder of social conditioning. More people watch the Super Bowl than vote for the president in this country. Many people are sending their children to fight a war with an enemy nobody has met. Even Galileo, under threat of death, had to confess to the Catholic Church that the world was the center of the universe. So what have we got here? We have a lot of pain and a lot of misunderstanding.

I want to tell you a story. I was once in a very heated disagreement with my family about my books. I thought they were good, and they said they weren't. I had a girlfriend who thought the world of my work, so I ended up on her couch at 10:30 PM, and she let me watch the movie *Whale Rider*. The story is about a young woman learning to communicate with whales, or nature. Of course by the end of the film, she was riding the whale. I looked at my friend, and she told me, "I want to ride whales." I said, "I want to talk to animals." Not to sound cliché, but the moment I said that I realized something. I realized I wanted to do more than talk with animals. I wanted to discover nature and always be connected with it. In that moment it was so clear to me that the greatest thing one person or humanity can achieve is a connection to nature. That was the night I designed my holistic health pyramid. It has seven levels: breathing, sleeping, hydration, attitude, nutrition, fitness, and the crowning achievement of a connection to nature. They are the way and the path out of pain. I was certain I'd figured out something remarkable, and it moved me. I woke up the next morning with a very light heart.

This is one way to understand pain and how to pull it out of ourselves or release it. Overcoming pain is the ambition of the soul, I think. Unseen pain is the most powerful pain in our lives. There is a true line of least resistance, and that is what nature, the wolves, the birds, and the dogs understand. There is also the broken line of least resistance: insomnia, addiction, bad diet, hubris, and shallow breathing. Today we're going to talk about how to fix this pain and how to reconnect with nature. Good afternoon.

PAIN II

"Imagine if failing students in school were systematically eaten by passing students. Imagine if our war generals wept and trembled when soldiers were lost, or if sex resulted in one woman eating another man."

If you could spend seven days working on the line of least resistance resolving your pain, would you commit to that week if it meant one thousand days of joy, or would you continue a broken line of resistance, a habitual addictive lack of exercise, a lack of nutrition, a lack of connection to nature, and use of alcohol, drugs, and cigarettes? What line would you pursue if you were given the chance to resolve your own pain for a solid week?

As I've explained, other creatures of the world have a fundamentally different relationship to pain than human beings, and it's helpful to take another perspective on what adversity and pain are all about, even if it's from an animal or plant. Earlier I mentioned that a mother bird will weep and tremble if she loses a chick or an egg and that a wolf will lead a stationary life in a dark cave for several weeks in order to heal a broken leg. Were you aware that shark babies, when living inside their mothers, are actually forced to eat and kill each other, usually leaving only two or three left? That's nature for you. Certain species of pinecone and pine tree only release their precious seeds during the intense heat of forest fires, so even in death, nature promotes life. In fact, Rupert Sheldrick helped to discover these exact same phenomena in plant cells. When plant cells die, they stimulate more growth through hormone release and thus more cells and then more death and then more cells. There are mother spiders that allow their children to consume their own bodies after birth, and there are female praying mantises that literally eat their mate after sex.

So what is the point? Nature and all of its creatures never perpetuate their own losses. In fact, when was the last time you ever saw the garbage of nature? You never have. Nature never wastes, and in fact, nature is self-corrective. Its creatures will self-select out of the food chain and even out of the gene pool. Ethnobiology is the study of such activity. How can a humble prairie dog sacrifice its own life so that a predator will not tamper with the colony? That kind of turns survival of the fittest on its belly when you think about it, and yet, this is true. Imagine if failing students in school were systematically eaten by passing students. Imagine if our war generals wept and trembled when soldiers were lost, or if sex resulted in one woman eating another man.

Nature can manage pain effectively. It can learn from pain how to survive. For nature's creatures, pain is a part of life, a challenge in growth. Human beings, we often shrink away from a situation that could imply suffering. Nature does not perpetuate its pain or loss. Nature is self-correcting, so why aren't we that way? I'll tell you why. Fundamentally, human beings have lost the value of new experience and traded in their pleasure for recycling old experiences again and again. Hindus call it the Wheel of Karma, and we all know people who are stuck in their comfort zones with their routines. They go to their nine to five jobs, own a few shiny things, sleep in or step out on the weekends in the same crowd, and live their lives on repeat, experiencing the same painful moments again and again, while the old pleasures slowly fade, just like they are supposed to.

Nature, on the other hand, does not recycle old pain and only thrives on new challenges. Salmon travel around the whole world. Birds do as well. In fact, many creatures see more of the world than an average human being. Children should be included in this as well. Children are all about learning and riding into new experiences. A young child is very much like a scientist. You've seen children pull the tail on a cat or dog or pull on their mother's hair. When they do this, they want to see what happens. This impulse for the unknown, the new, is so much a part of life. If you're true to this creative impulse, I'd say you're living on the line of least resistance. Your connection to nature is about jumping off the wheel of karma and onto this line, this newness, this unknown circumstance that is always present. Bob Dylan once said he who isn't busy being born is busy dying. This is sort of like saying nature is always busy being born. Pain is really a comfort zone thing, and it's an addiction. When we engage in an activity again and again and expect the same pleasure, the same result, we are putting ourselves in harm's way. That can apply to many things in a person's life—a relationship, an addiction, a motivating factor for success. I tell you, it's everywhere, but here's what you can do. The moment you feel that familiar sense of pain and ask yourself what's the matter, remember to also ask yourself, what's the *anti*matter—meaning, what have I been resisting all of this time to experience this same familiar pain again and again? How can I break down this resistance and discover what it really is? Most importantly, how can I live along the line of least resistance? If you ask yourself what's the matter, what's the antimatter, what is the broken line, and what is the line of least resistance, it will just come down to a single decision.

Gandhi once had to have surgery to remove his appendix, but he did not want to be put to sleep. In fact, what he decided to do was to let them remove the organ while he was still awake, and while he was awake, he was chatting, very friendly, with the crowd. That, to me, is a clear example of the kind of power nature offers when you remove the factors in your life that give resistance—not the factors that give pain, the factors that give *resistance*. There is a tremendous difference between the two. Releasing pain requires you to live through it, so you have to be brave and bold enough to look at its face, feel it, and surrender it. The desire to release your pain must be equally intense as the pain itself. Equal amounts, that's what I've learned. If you don't manage your inner pain, it will accumulate. The art of overcoming adversity is a sacred art. Obviously, in our world, it is not widely understood. It's the reason I decided to draw the line of least resistance down my holistic pyramid. In order to maximize the holistic health pyramid potential, draw a line from the top straight to the bottom. That way, you have the shortest distance between a connection to nature and your breath. Do you follow?

I've looked at ways to help us conquer pain, and I will continue to look and create better ways to explain the value of this idea. For today, the adversity should be a great contemplation. You know our forefathers had plenty of adversity. Actually, our ancestors went out to buy fur coats with a knife. Today, there is no shortage of resistance out there, so let the journey begin. In every matter, there is antimatter. Within every sorrow lives an unseen pearl, and you can find it if you bring yourself into honesty. Will it be worth living clean and healthy for seven days if it can bring one thousand days of joy? The answer is all up to you.

DID YOU KNOW THE
MAGIC OF NATURE?

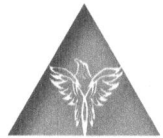

*"Did you know that when you light a candle in space,
you get a spherical-shaped candle flame?"*

The information I'm going to share with you today is sourced from several books, which I will list throughout the reading and at the end. Did you know that the oldest recorded woman in the world, Jeanne Calment, smoked cigarettes until she was 119, drank wine every night, and cussed like a sailor? Did you know that when an underwater air bubble is hit by a high-powered sound wave and explodes, it emits light? Scientists don't know why, but it does. Did you know that the aurora borealis, those lights in the sky near the North and South Poles, actually make noise? We do not understand why that happens either. However, we do know sound cannot travel through space. Did you know that the Earth is not a sphere but is actually flattened at either pole? It also bulges a bit at the midsection, or the equator. Did you know that plants can think? A man named Clive Backster once used a polygraph lie detector on his dragon tree, and it measured very astute reactions to being dunked underwater and soaked in hot coffee. Reactions from the dragon tree were recorded *before* the soaking and dunking took place. In fact, Backster found that the plants reacted the moment he made the mental decision to soak them. Did you know that Mr. Backster also used a polygraph on a store-bought, unfertilized chicken egg and, astonishingly, detected a faint pulsation? When opening the egg, it contained no circulatory function of any kind.

Did you know that a scientist named Rupert Sheldrake once used lots of hidden cameras to study the behavior of dogs and found, that without a doubt, domesticated dogs visibly prepare when the owner even makes the decision to return home? Did you know that Timiryazev Academy of Sciences once used an extremely sensitive electronic instrument that revealed the "scream" of a barley sprout when its roots where plunged into hot water? The article was in *Pravda,* the Russian newspaper read by millions, and remains available. Did you know that Kazakh scientists used the system developed by Pavlov, for dogs, on philodendrons? Each time the scientist placed a mineral ore next to the plant, it received an electric shock, and after several shocks for conditioning, the same plant would register elevated readings on a polygraph and electrocenograph when the mineral was put beside it. According to the famous contemporary plant biologist C. Louis Kervran, corn grown in a field of magnesium-depleted soil, in a controlled experiment, revealed that more magnesium was in the corn itself than in the soil. He concluded that plants have the ability to transmute basic elements. He also discovered, in another controlled experiment, that human beings on potassium-minimized diets working long hours in the desert appeared to convert a small portion of sodium into potassium. Dr. A.R. Bailey in 1972 placed two plants in an artificially lit greenhouse with the same humidity, temperature, light, and carefully controlled lack of water, and when he decided to water one plant, the other plant responded by generating measurable voltages, as though the plant was screaming out for water.

In the movie *Something Unknown Is Doing We Don't Know What* by Rene Scheltema, a group of common people are asked to look at a series of images, mostly landscapes, with graphic and violent images dispersed through the sequence. The people were hooked up to an instrument that could measure the dilation of the pupil and adrenal stress factors. What they discovered was interesting. Milliseconds *before* the graphic images were displayed, the body responded against hostility. The same did not happen with the serene and peaceful images. In this same film, random number generators hooked up all over the world recorded more of the same numbers during New Year's Eve, and especially one minute before the new year at 11:59 PM, than at any other time in the year. This occurred sequentially in every time zone.

Did you know the Nobel-Prize-winning great Bengali scientist Sir Jagadis Chandra Bose once published an eight-thousand-page column of 315 separate experiments on "plant response as a means of physiological investigation"? The experiments showed that plants, in their movement growth, actually absorb energy from their surroundings. One reviewer said, "The student of plant physiology who has some acquaintance with the main classical ideas of his subject will feel at first extreme bewilderment as he peruses this book."

Did you know that famous author George Bernard Shaw, while visiting Jagadis Bose, looked through a microscope at a cabbage leaf magnified 100 million times and quote "observed the cabbage leaf going through violent paroxysms as it was scalded to death." George Bernard Shaw later remained vegetarian but became an antivivisectionist as well, and he dedicated his own collected works to Bose, inscribing them "From the least to the greatest living biologist." Did you know that in 1968 Dorothy Retallack and biology professor Francis F. Broman had the novel idea to grow plants next to two forms of music, a classical radio station that played Brahms, Schubert, Haydn, and eighteenth and nineteenth century scores and a Denver rock-and-roll radio station with extremely percussive rock music from Vanilla Fudge, Hendrix, and Led Zeppelin. They found not only that classical music helped the plants grow 30 percent faster, but also that the plants actually grew toward the speakers. Even more interesting is that when classical music plants were put up against Hindu music, Ravi Shankar, sitarists, and even choral preludes to Johann Sebastian Bach, the plants were more inspired and grew more toward the sitar and Bach collection. Some of those plants bent at an angle in excess of 60 degrees, and one plant almost took hold of the speaker itself.

Did you know that Dr. George Starr White, author of *Cosmo Electric Culture*, discovered that metals such as iron and tin could facilitate plant growth if bright pieces were dangled from fruit trees. As he put it, "At first my wife would not let me hang the balls on the plants because she said it looked ridiculous. But when fifteen potted tomatoes hung with balls started to ripen in the cold, inclement weather long before those of any other grower, she allowed me to continue."

Did you know that when you light a candle in space, you get a spherical-shaped candle flame? According to NASA, the microgravity applications division, Project Candle Flame, this occurs because without gravity, convection current cannot occur, so we are left with a big blue ball of fire. Did you know?

Did you know a whole range of studies was performed on the Fox0 gene? Interest in this very unique genome began when marine biologists identified a hydra (sea creature) that does not appear to age. According to *Science Daily*, "The freshwater polyp hydra does not show any signs of aging and appears to be immortal." Why? After much research, it was determined that this creature possessed an inordinate amount of stem-cell activity. For the most part, the immortality gene caused this stem-cell activity.

Did you know Duke University has also identified the Fox0 gene? Did you know that modern human beings possess dormant Fox0 genes? Clearly, we were designed to live longer than seventy-three years. Stem-cell therapy and research are the prima materia of future medicine.

Do you know the 914 pages of a long-forgotten seminal work in archeology called *Forbidden Archeology: The Hidden History of the Human Race*? Michael Cremo wrote it. It is his life's work and details seven-foot-tall women with red hair who wear plaid and were buried on the Silk Road from East China to Persia. It reveals the forgotten exhibits of larger skeletons in New York City's Museum of Natural History. These exhibits are real and only date back to early last century. Some say there are still giant femur bones of human beings buried in the basement of the Natural History Museum.

Hey, did you know that our domesticated animals will chew on grass if sick? Did you know there are migrating goats in South America that trek hundreds of miles toward the ocean at the end of each spring season to lick the salt off the rocks? More sodium in their body helps to retain moisture throughout those hot South American summers. Did you know that in the 1960s, wild coyotes in Los Angeles were threatened by the quickened growth of modern civilization? Animal scientists noted a very peculiar phenomenon: the coyotes tripled their birthrate, and 75 percent of their litters were female. Did you know the coyotes never had a conference; they did not use phones. Did you know that salmon travel upstream to lay their eggs in the same spot where they were born? Marine biologists have noted that even if an old stream has dried up, salmon will have prior knowledge of an alternate route and use it on their journey home.

Did you know that animals can detect changes in the weather? Worms flee rising groundwater. Birds respond to changes in air pressure well before bad weather occurs; they have actually been seen to prepare for storms. Bears have been observed to flee before severe earthquakes, sometimes even coming out of hibernation. Did you know? In Florida, researchers monitoring tagged sharks have reported that they escape to deeper water just before a big hurricane arrives. "I think these animals are more attuned to their environment than we give them credit for," says Michelle Heupel, a scientist at the Mote Marine Laboratory that worked on the shark study.

Did you know that a small handful of what scientists are calling "dark matter," "mirror matter," or "antimatter" contains enough energy to power the whole world for several years? Did you know that another word for "levitation" is "electrostatic propulsion," according to Nick Cook, author of *The Hunt for Zero Point*? Did you know that the mathematical proportions of the arm-to-wing spans, stamen-to-stalk, curve of a seashell, petal to flower, and arms of the galaxy are all one mathematical ratio called the "golden ratio" or the "golden section," a proportion universally present in nature? Did you know that pleurisy flowers and mullein leaves, two outstanding herbs to improve respiratory function, have typically been found growing in tobacco fields of Kentucky? In fact, these lung savers are always the most common "weed" around. Did you know that Leonardo da Vinci drew *Sketches of Aeroship*, and it looks exactly the same as a flying saucer or UFO? Did you know that the soul has been photographed leaving the body as a white mist from the center of the chest? Did you know that during what we call multiple personality disorder the human body can literally transform, vision can be altered, and allergies can actually disappear? Did you know that the placebo effect is so powerful it can account for 30 percent of the success of any so-called drug, even a sugar pill? Did you know it is possible to fool a lie detector test with focused attention? Did you know that children under the age of three can regrow the top part of their fingers if they happen to be cut off? Did you know that according to MRIs, most people are using less than 5 percent of their own brains? Did you know that most people grow less than 15 percent of the hair on their heads? Did you know that most people use less than 40 percent of their lung capacity? Did you know that most people use less than half of their vocal cord capacity? Did you know that science has not conclusively found the seat of consciousness within the brain, and that perhaps the brain can be likened to a reducing valve? Did you know that a few days after death, each and every cell in the corpse explodes? It's called "corruption."

Did you know nobody understands why lightning has such an incongruent or unset path? Did you know that the arms industry and the pharmaceutical industry are the largest industries in the world? Did you know that scientists have validated that near-death experiences are actually valid, according to a new study in the British medical journal *Lancet*, which researched and reviewed over 300 near-death experiences? Did you know that science recently discovered the god particle, and that it's shaped like a spiral? Did you know that there are more stars in the galaxies around us than there are grains sands on all the beaches in the world? Did you know that the human eye has a blind spot? Daniel J. Boorstin once said, "The greatest obstacle to discovery is not ignorance, but the illusion of knowledge." Did you know that most people don't know that they don't know what they don't know?

Did you know that Ronald Reagan confessed to a reporter that the CIA used professional remote viewers to find criminals? A remote viewer is a person who can see into the future or at any distance using his or her mind. Did you know that every time you sit on the ground, you are actually levitating? There is an electromagnetic force between you and the Earth all the time; although it may be a very small space, it is still there. Did you know that sea salt has been proposed to solve the world's hunger problems, according to R. Maynard Murray and his book *Sea Energy Agriculture*? Did you know that garlic, oregano oil, basil, and elderberry have been proven to help fight cancer? Did you know that Germany has found more than one so-called cure for AIDS? Did you know that Magic Johnson privately takes his vacations in Germany?

Irreducible Mind, by Edward and Emily Kelly
Golden Thread magazine, February–April 2002
The Seven Fundamentals of Longevity
The Secret Life of Plants by Christopher Bird
Food is Medicine by Dr. Brain Clement

THE ORDER OF
ELIMINATION

"Why is simple efficiency such a struggle for humankind? How come we can't help but leave our shit all over the place?"

Today we're going to talk about your tears. Your sweat. Your urine. And the wonderful world of your bowels. So for part of our show, we're going to be talking about human waste; human elimination. Many of us have an issue with it. It's not a charming topic, but it is a natural function of your body. You know, this aversion to human waste is a deep subject. How deep? I hardly need a single statistic to tell you that human beings are the most wasteful creatures on Earth or that our waste has long been unbearable to other creatures on Earth, not to mention ourselves. Why is simple efficiency such a struggle for humankind? How come we can't help but leave our shit all over the place? Because the average person today is not a master of order.

Order is the next topic today. Order in life is so vitally important. With no order, nobody gets healthy and maintains their health for any length of time. Without order, there is no harmony or balance. So we'll have to talk about cleaning our closets, skin cleansing, bowel cleansing, mental exercises, and taking the time to shed our old skin. Hey, maybe when we shed our old skins, they will be biodegradable! That would be a nice way to help complete nature's cycle, wouldn't it? Whether it comes to peak performance, healing, or weight loss, you should know that it is always essential to have your ducks in order. Usually, maintaining order in their lives is the first and foremost problem people have. After all, most people are at work to simply survive. If I may, I'd like to tell you a story about a Zen master who was given three new students and taught them a lesson in what he called *intent* and *timing*.

He said to the students, "You will wash my clothes, cook my soup, tend to my garden, and build my fire until the day I see you are true masters. When you are, you will be ready to learn the great truths of the supernatural world and be enlightened."

Every day for three years the students toiled in his garden, slaved over his clothes, cooked his food, and built his fire. If the master noticed a spot on his robe, he pointed it out to them. When a student was late, he said, "You are a late student." When a student was not joyfully participating in his duties, he would say to him, "You, you are no master. You are a lazy duck."

For four more years, they continued performing the hard labor but never with zeal or precision. Then, one day, a student threw down his fire poker, leapt into the master's face, and screamed, "Master! Why, if you say that we are really so magical and supernatural, must we do all of these things?"

The master's face was unwavering as he said, "Alas student, when you learn how to do all of these things without waste, then you will understand exactly how magical you really are."

Did you know that the Nobel-Prize-winning scientist Alexis Carrel kept chicken heart cells alive in a Petri dish for more than twenty years just by removing their waste products and feeding them nutrients? Did you know that at the bottom of the ocean floor, manganese rocks are expelled from volcanoes that actually clean the ocean? Did you know that rain water is 1 percent hydrogen peroxide, and that it disinfects our soil and crops so that they may grow and so creatures like you and me can eat them? Have you ever seen nature's trash? Have you ever lifted up a fallen tree and found thousands of creatures alive and well? Nature has no trash. Nature does not waste.

Picasso once said, "Art is the elimination of the unnecessary." Why would you cleanse lungs that will eventually smoke fifty more packs of dirty cigarettes? Why would you clean your gut if you never planned to eat healthier? Why would you box with the champ with both hands tied behind your back? Who is the champ? It's nature and the connection existing between nature and yourself. To quote Aristotle, "Excellence is a habit." Therefore, before you take that step of cleaning out your body and keeping it well, let's talk about what you can do to assume control over your mental habits. We can start with five synergistic exercises of my own design.

Exercise 1. Recite classic poetry and literature with feeling. This exercise is great for the shy person and is not complicated. It will activate your emotional sensor. It will keep you comfortable on your feet. Read poetry and prose that inspires you aloud. You do not have to do it in front of anybody. Reading and expressing emotion with literature is a safe and comfortable way to break through your inhibitions. It can also be a great exercise in improving your articulation. It may also help you get through your day at work by helping you learn to live inside your imagination. Let this exercise strengthen your diction and character. It can help open you up. Stand up in your room and walk around, get animated, be present and act out an incredible story. I know you will have an incredible time trying this exercise. It stimulates the imagination, concentration, and emotions. It will be worth doing if you are feeling locked up inside. I recommend you read the works of William Shakespeare, because his treatment of the English language set a standard for all future wordsmiths. The ways in which we speak are very much influenced by his work.

Exercise 2. Trace in peroxide. Now that you have read and activated your imagination and emotional core for the better part of the morning, you should be in better shape. Your goal is now to strengthen your concentration or mental acuity. In other words, you must strengthen your mind by improving focus and strengthening the nervous system. Do this by taking an hour to trace great works of art very slowly while soaking your feet in a watery hydrogen peroxide tub. This exercise synergistically fosters razor-sharp mental focus and deep oxygenation of the brain. A foot bath soothes the nervous system and greatly improves mental strength. You will notice that soaking your feet in hydrogen peroxide improves your ability to breath, trace, and focus. That is because large amounts of oxygen are being absorbed through the skin, into the blood, and safely being delivered into the brain. After you select the work that you want to trace, remember to be completely and utterly uninterrupted, active in the moment, and breathing rhythmically. When you trace, keep your head and body relaxed and still. Do not get involved with completing the work. Learn to focus in the moment. Be present and enjoy the process.

Exercise 3. Write down what you want. Now it's time to use your heightened imagination and focus for something special. Have you ever taken the time to sit and think about what has been on your mind? Have you ever faced your inner desires through contemplation or meditation? Do you allow yourself time for learning about the things that you would personally like to achieve in your life?

Contemplation is a lost art. The best way to reprioritize and clean up your act is to spend several hours writing down what you want. This exercise will help to retrain your mind to discover what you need at any given moment. Obviously your greatest need must be your greatest priority. Hour after hour of writing your desires will help you to discover your own self-contrived shortcomings. This identification is very important. Either before or after you write down the desire, start identifying what you lack. As you write more and more of what you desire or what you perceive to be lacking, you will then feel an added spaciousness to your heart. When face-to-face with your own shortcomings, you will realize that subconscious feelings of something lacking really do not serve you in the moment. Go ahead and dispatch your feelings of lacking and limitation. Focusing on your self contrived lack will help you realize how meaningless and impractical it really is to you. In my opinion, there is no greater tool for healing the body, mind, and spirit than sitting down for one to four hours and writing page after page of your desires as they come to you.

Exercise 4. Take out the trash. When you have a clear idea of what you want, you gain insight into the myriad ways in which you have attempted to fill the void, the emptiness of lacking in the past. They are old ways. Often enough they do not serve us well. It's true that old habits die hard, so now it's time to physically clean up the past. Engage in cleaning from the ground up. Clean your room and your closets. Move items into another room or donate your clothes. You could have a yard sale or put things in storage. If you are going to prioritize your actions and your mind, you will need to clean up and prioritize the space where you spend the most time. You do not have to make your room sparse or Zen-like; however, there is one rule to follow. Remove anything from your room that does not make you happy. This practice will help you form more intelligent desires and healthy boundaries in your life. Keeping your space clean and orderly on a daily basis will help continue to reinforce those healthy boundaries you create. If you stick with the practice, you may one day discover an openness and extra space in your heart. By attending to your space, you might find yourself becoming more creative, insightful, and logical. This is because you won't be reactivating old habits built on false and primitive needs. With a new desire to live, you can begin to recreate your life.

Exercise 5. Write a schedule for your day. Now that you have activated your emotional core, heightened your focus, addressed your self-contrived shortcomings by determining what you want out of life, and cleared the path for a new life, it's time to write a schedule for your day. This last exercise will help propel all that you have learned out into the world, bringing your personal growth beyond the walls of your living space. Imagine what it would be like to write a schedule for your day before doing any of these previous exercises. Writing a truly superb daily schedule requires knowledge of your desires, concentration, imagination, and commitment. It will steer you away from reactivating old habits. It will bring you closer to the things you desire most in your life. Once again, this is the accumulation of all that you have done up until this point. Keep yourself on track. Make your schedule as detailed as possible. At eight o'clock in the morning you may brush your teeth. At eight-twenty you may stretch. At eight-thirty you might eat breakfast. Perhaps you do not know what you will be doing at four o'clock in the afternoon. Write "miscellaneous time, place, and event" and wait to see what four o'clock will bring you, or write "controlled chaos" or insert breathing exercises into your day or other activities you have been waiting to try. Use that intensified imagination.

When it comes to building health back into the body, there are many talented medicine men and women out there who can help you. Likewise, there are many talented pharmaceutical sales representatives and salesmen of all kinds. In the sales-driven world, it is better to add to your medicine chest than subtract—and, obviously, a self-destructive habit. In the order of elimination, it's much better to subtract than to add. Many people will suggest you take their little blue pill and that it resolves all ills and brings everything back into its place, but I'll tell you, the order of wholeness begins with the order of elimination. Always take the red pill instead and eliminate toxic beverages, foods, habits, and addictions. Eliminate immoderate and imbalanced people, places, things, and events. Work toward simplicity and take back your power, and you will quickly understand that the greatest medicine is not a water fast or a master cleanse but a fast of the mind: a fast from self-deceit, wastefulness, and obvious destruction.

So, for the body there are five avenues of elimination: the skin, the bowels, the breath, the urine, and the tear. For the skin, I recommend infrared saunas, skin brushing, and sea salt/baking soda baths each night for four or five nights. Run a hot bath and add one cup of sea salt with one-half cup of baking soda. Bathe for thirty minutes, max. For the bowel, I can recommend many things. Some of the most overlooked methods are toilet yoga, polenta, or cornmeal and my lemon pollen honey hot tea. "Toilet yoga" is just discovering what posture or postures work for you on the john. Frequently people do well with their knees above their waistline. Some of the best breathing exercises for respiratory elimination are slow breathing, limbic breathing, alternate nostril breathing, or any yogic technique. Visit a yoga class to find out how to do them.

The next avenue of elimination is the urine. For this, working with diuretic herbs like hibiscus and nettle are really wonderful. One day a week without solid food, eating only soups and vegetable juices instead, is a great idea also. There is a fifth avenue of elimination, and it's the human tear—yes, water, human, emotional tears. Chemically, emotional tears are very different from ordinary human tears. We can all agree that they release enough burdens when wept sincerely. They can be considered the fifth avenue of proper elimination.

There are also five mental exercises that will help you to get into the secure place for elimination. All I have left is to ask, what is the one thing in your life that, if given up, would make the largest positive impact on your life? What could you surrender? What could you sacrifice? You can call in and share or think about it. Thank you for listening.

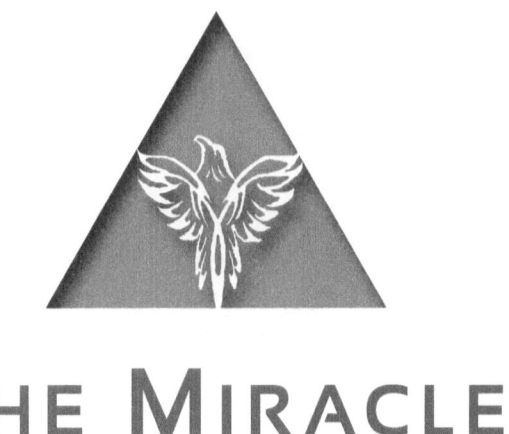

THE MIRACLE

"One of the greatest Americans in recent history, William Cooper, said it best I think. Anyone keeping secrets obviously has something to hide."

Today we are going to try something different. Today I'm going to start by asking you a very unusual question, and I'd like you to participate and form an answer for yourself. Okay? Here it goes. In the studio at this very moment I'm holding an object in the palm of my hand. What am I holding? Beyond what I've told you, I won't give you any more information. I'd like you to take a stab, a guess, a nonsense answer. I want a nonsense answer. That means I don't want you to touch, taste, see, or hear your way over here. Use the "Force." Come up with a strong intuitive feeling, and please remember it. We're going to perform a miracle today.

If your answer was a book or a blue book, I would like you to pour a glass of cold water and throw it on your face. You've got it. The book is called *Psychic Warrior* by David Morehouse. It's about the CIA's remote viewing program. As a remote viewer, Morehouse gave vital and accurate information to our military during the Gulf War. He also uncovered a few sinister plots that I won't divulge; rather, you should read it and find out for yourself. What I just asked you to do with the book is called a remote view. The former president of the United States, Ronald Reagan, admitted to the secret project's existence in an interview after his second term.

Today I'm not going to discuss the veracity of occult knowledge, but its history, purpose, and methodology and why we should pay attention to those forgotten souls who have always laid it on the line. If you think about it, most of us source our information from TV, government officials, scientists, health gurus, doctors, and authors, but if we were to take a step backward for a moment and examine human history, you'd find an impressive and large amount of information sourced from "occult" or "unknown" origins. Aside from the great oracle at Delphi, Nostradamus, and John Dee, close and personal friend of Elizabeth I, the Old Testament is quite loaded with psychic talent. Abraham heard voices, went into trances, and had meaningful visions. Daniel, who fell into the lion's den, was a seer as well. Joseph was strongly precognitive and could interpret dreams. Olam was clairvoyant and clairaudient, and so was Gideon. The "Seer" tradition includes Pythagoras, Plotinus, Jesus, Socrates, the apostle Paul, and even Apollonius of Tyana. In keeping with these very old traditions, religious groups and new-age groups and even cult factions today have organizational structures; there is a medium or a channel and then there are the listeners. This is an old story being refreshed by new-age organizations, so they're really old age organizations if you think about it.

Today I'd like to talk about five of the most prolific seers of the modern day, and I'd like to tell you how each of them embodied different approaches to the same fantastic remarkable goal and enlightened selfhood and a stronger connection to nature. Those people I'd like to talk with you about are Edgar Cayce, J.Z. Knight, Arthur Ford, John of God, and Elwood Babbitt. Perhaps in seven thousand years these will be the players in a future old testament, and maybe after I acquaint you with the scope and beauty of their work, their tireless hours of service, and their unsung contributions to the world today, you will be inspired to pick up one of their autobiographies. I hope so.

As Shakespeare once wrote in *Hamlet*, there is more on heaven and Earth than is dreamt of in your philosophy, Horatio. According to Mr. Elwood Babbitt, Shakespeare and others had much more to say on the subject of reincarnation. Elwood Babbitt, upon whom the film *Free Spirits* is based, was an undeniably talented transmedium who served as a spiritual bridge for many famous historical personalities, including Albert Einstein, Sigmund Freud, William Wordsworth, Adlai Stevenson, Abraham Lincoln, John F. Kennedy, Louis Armstrong, Bishop Pike, and Mark Twain. Whether you're neophyte, skeptic, or seasoned veteran in the world of spirit communication, it cannot detract from Mark Twain's immortal sense of humor: "Well, I suppose I have to announce my identity. God knows why. Nobody will believe it, anyway. But I'm Mark Twain, Sam Clemens, old fool if you prefer. But I've been asked to come through this narrow canal once again into earth. And of course I made the trip once before between all the bumps and belches, and squelches from gastronomical odors that prevail in the birth cycle."

Elwood Babbitt has published books claiming to be in mediumship with Jesus of Nazareth and the lord god Vishnu. Regardless of his authenticity, Elwood Babbitt's manuscripts show a very advanced level of historical savvy, vocabulary, humor, and use of language. This next poem, from an unknown source, came through Mr. Babbitt on October 8, 1973, and it's been on my wall in the Phoenix Institute of Montclair for over five years. It's one of my favorite poems, actually:

> When in the dim beginning of the years
> God mixed in man the rapture and the tears
> And scattered through his brain the starry stuff,
> He said, "Behold, yet this is not enough,
> For I must test his spirit to make sure

That he can dare the vision and endure,
Leaving behind only a broken clue,
A crevice where the Glory glimmers through,
Leaving him in tragic loneliness to choose,
With all in life to win, or all in life to lose.

Our next medium is probably without a doubt the most well-known, the late Edgar Cayce. Mr. Cayce was a simple man, a photographer, a Christian who read his Bible once a year. Like many of the great mediums of the West, Cayce was forced into the world by an unseen hand if you will. Cayce was known to "speak on many subjects, from Atlantis, relationships, and natural health to giving the locations of missing persons and missing children, very often with dead-on accuracy. His recorded sessions fill an entire vault of books, and there are still people today who make it their job to sort and organize the Cayce readings, nearly forty years later. My grandfather, who was a Buddhist, read many of Edgar Cayce's books. Beginning when I was sixteen, I became acquainted with Cayce through my grandfather's hand-me-downs, and they bring back many wonderful memories for me. During the 1920s he gave people many remedies from olive oil, castor oil, and lemon juice to high-frequency violet rays. This made him known as the "father of holistic medicine." However, I would like to make it very clear that this was a title someone else applied to Edgar Cayce.

Edgar Cayce was as authentic as another prolific channel, J. Z. Knight, only Cayce never had the opportunity to be psychologically, physiologically, and scientifically tested like J. Z. Knight. Once during in his career, however, Cayce was arrested and brought to jail. He was physically frail as a person and was immediately cornered in a room with aggressive, strong criminals. What did he do? He began to very rapidly tell each of these strong criminals their reason for being incarcerated, the loved ones they had left behind, and their deepest, darkest secrets. What happened? The convicts were so impressed that he was unharmed and became the Virginia State Prison's unofficial local psychic, giving everyone free readings, and he developed a very kind and trustworthy reputation there. One might recall Daniel in the lion's den.

The next prophet of the day is the aforementioned Ms. J. Z. Knight. Of all the rarities in this strange realm, none is more gifted and unusual than J. Z. Knight and her unseen confidant Ramtha, the Enlightened One. Why? Knight is the only medium to have been rigorously tested by science, and the outcome of these tests has left an extraordinary mark on the scientific community. J. Z. Knight is the real deal. When channeling Ramtha, her eyes change color from blue to gray, her neck widens, her brainwaves drop immediately into the deepest delta state, and the new visitor, Ramtha, puts on an amazing show. It is not uncommon by any means to see the character who calls himself Ramtha, the Enlightened One speak on stage for over twenty hours without a break; to lift men three times J. Z. Knight's size and carry them across the room or a hall; to do back flips while dancing, accurately predicting the future, and delivering witticisms and inspiration; or simply performing miracles in the English language well beyond the ability of Elwood Babbitt.

> "Why do you not possess the power of regeneration of new tissue, new skin, new organ, new limb, and new body? What does the common humble salamander know that you don't know? What do fish know, special fish and frogs that you don't know that they can bury themselves from one season of birth of activity deep into the soft mud and quicksand of a river bed, going quickly, evaporating up and live there for lives in a catatonic dream, intact and

hibernating until after a 12-year drought or a 20-year drought and the rains come. And the rains begin to quench the dry earth and the riverbed nearly forgotten by a new generation that it ever was, suddenly from the high places in the land the water rushes from its tributaries and fills the riverbed with life-giving waters and over-night long hibernating seeds begin to grow and as the riverbed fills up the moisture is sunk into the depths where the slow marvelous creatures of nature are suddenly, with cool moisture, awakened from long slumber and made their ways to freshened springs and begin the birth and the regeneration of new generations and live life to its fullest, least it dry up again. What do these common, humble creatures possess that you do not possess?"

J. Z. Knight is unique in that she channels one being, Ramtha. It was Ramtha who actually coined the term *channel* and helped to distin-guish it from *mediumship*. A *channel* is someone who completely evac-uates the body, likened unto death, whereas a *medium* is someone with "one foot in each world', if you will. I've personally met Ramtha as well as J. Z. Knight, and I can say in all sincerity that no mere mortal could ever perform at the level that J. Z. Knight and Ramtha have for the past forty years. They are a gift to the world, in my humble opinion. Pick up the DVD *Create Your Day* and have a look yourself.

Another gift to the world is the humble and very sweet man they call John of God. John of God is based in Brazil and also claims to be a pure channel. He has, verifiably, performed healing miracles on a reg-ular basis and has become quite well known in South America. Part of what makes John of God fascinating is the way in which he performs the art of supernatural healing. He uses a knife. There are many videos on the Internet and DVDs about him, and you can watch him stick his knife deep into the eye or nose of a volunteer and then watch them throw away their reading glasses without bleeding. It's amazing!

The last modern-day seer of the day is Arthur Ford. Arthur Ford has largely been forgotten, but he deserves to be remembered. Arthur Ford was a brilliant author and channel who was made famous by Harry Houdini in the 1930s. He is the author of the book *Unknown but Known*, a wonderful little book detailing the history of seers and prophets of ancient and modern origin.

All of this exciting phenomena happening in our lifetime is exactly the kind of food for thought we need. When people continuously lose their connection to nature, there always has been and will be an occult force at work to fortify and reconnect us to that vital life force. It isn't as uncommon as you might have been led to believe. In fact, many of us have been led to believe otherwise and have been trained in the false catalog of superstition and unexamined ritual. Individuals like Edgar Cayce who dares to go out on a limb and meet challenge with truth and authority should be admired, because they represent the kind of audacity that Jesus or Buddha once had. Buddha was a prince who left his life and climbed over the walls of the city alone to walk into the forest and humbly, ultimately live one with God.

Jesus was also a seditious man who never compromised what he believed to be right. Was he a lover of nature? There is a story in the Bible that makes it perfectly clear that he was. He and his disciples were sleeping under a bridge beside a beautiful field of lilies. His disciples, who were probably hungry and uncomfortable sleeping on the good earth herself, said, "Shouldn't we find a better place?" Jesus said to them, "Do you see those lilies over there? King Solomon in all his glory could not wear a robe more beautiful than the lilies in the field." Enough said. Jesus was all about the connection to nature.

What does the word *occult* actually mean? It literally means "unknown or secret knowledge." It has also been defined as "secret teachings." In fact, the word *cult* is a derivation of *occult*, and its definition is "a group that keeps secret teachings or secret knowledge." In this classical definition, all people in organizations that keep classified information or secrets are occult organizations, and that includes the secret archives in Vatican City, the classified information of our government, corporations, and all cults that have secret branches. The word *occult* is also used to define human blood. In medicine, if one discovers a sort of unusual or different type of blood in a human being they call it "occult blood." The word *occult* is also used to describe the unknown actions of certain bacteria that are then called "occult bacteria." What is remarkable about the five individuals I've described is that there are hardly any secrets or occults in their work, so I find them worthy to promote and worthy to study. One of the greatest Americans in recent history, William Cooper, said it best I think: Anyone keeping secrets obviously has something to hide. The Cayce and Ramtha files combined could exceed the amount of information contained in fifty King James Bibles. Only an open society that is of the people and by the people with sincere intentions could create such a wonderful and accessible work of art.

THE FUTURE OF
HEALTH

"I would be remiss if I did not share this with people who could really, really use it."

I've met so many people who struggle with self-starting, getting their businesses together or taking care of their businesses, so in the past I've recommended reading autobiographies by people such as Nelson Mandel, Helen Keller, Malcolm X, and Benjamin Franklin. I've also recommended watching inspirational TED Talks, Upworthy videos, and other films like *It's a Wonderful Life*, *E. T. the Extra Terrestrial*, *Life is Beautiful*, *Forrest Gump*, or *To Kill a Mockingbird*. All of these can increase your will to live. I've also recommended a better diet, breathing exercises, and ways to get deeper rest. Once, I had the idea to open up a nondenominational will-to-live center so people could keep their inspirational fires burning, and I still want to pursue this venture in the near future, but today I'm going to talk about something that inspires me.

When I was thirteen, my mother came down with a severe case of viral meningitis that had her bedridden for four months. It was bad. Each week she had headaches and double and then triple vision, and by the third month my father, who feared the worst, brought her to our beach house on Fire Island, where she could rest by the calm sound of the ocean. At the time, our days were spent helping her, and I will never forget the amount of drugs she had been prescribed that were sitting on her bedside table. I remember at least seven medications there.

Usually the drugs were there to counteract the terrible side effects of other drugs. This was a very rough time for my whole family. One day I told her, "Mom, you should swim in the ocean. Today. It will help you feel better." My mother's tired eyes widened. She was given to trusting her intuition, so she put on a bathing suit, and I made the slow walk to the ocean with her. It was a calm day on the shore, and I remember in the very beginning my mother just stood in the ocean, letting the waves move over her abdomen while she did not move at all. Later, perhaps ten minutes later, she began to gently swim. For an hour my mother swam there. Her nose was running; the ocean was detoxifying her respiratory system, her brain, her eyes, clearing her throat. She experienced no headache in the ocean—none at all. She told me she wanted to come back the next day, and we did. The second day she swam in a wetsuit for twenty minutes. She did the same thing on the third, fourth, and fifth days. On day six, she stopped all of her medication, because swimming in the ocean just seemed to work better for her. It did, and so she swam. She swam for the next week until she was completely, totally restored in her health.

I'm reminded of how simple it can be. How often do we imagine our challenges so daunting and horrifying that we could never face them, and weeks go by and it suddenly dawns on us, "here! This is what I've really been missing". It's my job to help people with this common conflict. Human beings tend to complicate things. I try to simplify them. The work is not hard work, but the effort can be challenging. It's all about thinking new thoughts, thinking differently, coming up with ideal original approaches. Today the future of natural health care inspires me. I'm inspired by those special five-star treatments that are still available to the American public: intravenous ozone therapy, photoluminescent therapy, peroxide drips, infrared saunas, cold lasers, and hypothermic treatments. I'm telling you, if you're in trouble and looking for the ocean, you can start with that and then try these other treatments. If you are interested, watch Gary Null's *Ozone Therapy: The Miracle Medicine* and read William Douglas Campbell's *Into the Light* and understand that there is more on Earth than is dreamt of in medical philosophy. That's how it is. I would be remiss if I did not share this with people who could really, really use it, so take my advice. I swear it's made of silver and gold. Go support the brave pioneers in medicine who are paving the way for what will become scientific revolution in years ahead. Do your own research; visit clinics; ask questions; seek second, third, and fourth opinions. You should know that many of these same treatments are used successfully in countries such as Japan and Germany where overall health and longevity soars when compared with America. No one knows all the answers; however, there are more out there. I hope you find them.

SENSORY DEPRIVATION
& RESTORATION

"In every case, from the shamans in the southwest and voodoo doctors of Haiti to the magi and healers of India, there is a specific course of action that is supposed to bring out the soul, the psyche, the supernatural mind, the true healer within all of us. It's the saint in the cave. It's the blindfold. It's the Indian in the hole covered in darkness until the day he discovers his soul. That is sensory deprivation, and it has a long legacy of miracles attached to it."

I once met an autistic boy who visited my office for a foot bath. His mother doubted whether I could administer an ionic foot bath to him for any significant period of time, because all day he constantly moved and could not seem to get control of himself. I felt an enormous amount of compassion for the young man, because I too know what it's like not to be in control of one's faculties. I knew what to do, however. I observed his mother insisting that he relax, to no avail. She went outside to make a long phone call. I stayed with him. I made eye contact with him, politely grinned, and began a long series of deep and powerful breaths. I observed that the young man showed no interest in following any instructions. If I breathed, he breathed. If I spoke, he spoke. If I stood up, he stood up. He was a great imitator. Later, I learned he was a musical savant and incredibly talented drummer. I led him through a series of powerful breaths, then a series of short, slow breaths; followed by a series of limbic exhales; followed by a series of powerful athletic breaths; followed by a series of alternate nostril breaths; followed by a series of blind bumblebee breaths; followed by a series of fire breaths; followed by a series of quick exhales; followed by a series of slow exhales. Within the span of twenty minutes, he and I were like two young dragons. He kept his feet still on the foot bath the entire time. I have never met anyone who could follow my instructions perfectly without being taught. His body, like mine, hungered for atmosphere, for air. He was a sensitive young man. He could feel that primal need for air. Toward the end, I found the change in his behavior entirely obvious. When his mother returned, I made sure she saw us breathing, and her son felt proud to show her what he had learned. He looked calm, collected, and finally attentive to people. To say his mother looked shocked would be an understatement. Both felt happy to have visited me. My doors have been and always will be open to them. I instructed his mother to stop using the words relax, calm down, or be quiet. Instead I suggested she replace those words with *breathe, breathe, good job, you can do it, breathe slowly,* and *very good, breathe.* This seemed to help their relationship tremendously. I also instructed her to breathe with him for ten to thirty minutes a day while following several of the techniques I've written in my third book, *The Seven Fundamentals of Longevity and the Holistic Health Pyramid.* The word *psyche* in Greek means soul and breath. They are the same word. It takes great willpower to discover this thing that we call the soul. Everyone is blessed with big lungs, and if you know how to use them, they can clear the path of the psyche.

I told you this story because there is really no greater medicine than a sharp and focused mind and a billowing lung. All we really need is enough inspiration to begin to breathe. There are two great stories on the healing power of breath that come to mind. One was done by Dr. Majid Ali and the other by Kamal Matiato. You can find Dr. Majid Ali's study on the Internet. He instructed nearly thirty people to do slow, deep breathing for five minutes and measured their blood pressures, heart rates, and breaths per minute. He found that some people saved over ten thousand breaths per day because they stopped breathing shallow, quick breaths. He found their blood pressures dropped to twenty to thirty points in only five minutes. My father, who has had issues with blood pressure, experienced this benefit firsthand.

Kamal Mattal set up an experiment in New Delhi where an entire building was given eight indoor plants per person. The found that air quality, human productivity, and blood oxygen levels improved and energy costs were reduced. It came to be the healthiest building in New Delhi. Incidents of asthma reduced by 9 percent, respiratory conditions by 34 percent, and headaches by 24 percent. Dr. Alexander Beddoe determined that 80 percent of human energy is derived not from food and water but from the air itself. This is why I spend so much time breathing and teaching people how to do it better. I used to have people perform five minutes of strong breathing exercises and then throw a blindfold on them and lay them down on a soft infrared heating mat under a bamboo pyramid. I turn on several air purifiers and aromatherapy and then play the 1812 Overture. I still do that. I also created the concept of the salt tent, which basically is a tent filled with sea salt in which you lie down and breathe. It's sort of like replicating the salt cave experience, only you can do it at home. I'm a very big fan of hydrogen peroxide baths, breathing garlic vapors, limbic breathing, Fenugreek, chlorella, all the beautiful things that help you reconnect with the psyche. The psyche, according to Greek lore, was difficult to discover because the body—its neuroses, its appetites, its passions—would tend to steer the soul off course. It's said in Fido by Socrates that the senses do not grasp reality in any way. No two people will ever hear or see the same thing in an identical way.

This leads me to my main point in all of this. Today I'm very interested in sensory deprivation and sensory restoration. I've discovered and studied ancient esoteric science. In every case, from the shamans in the Southwest and voodoo doctors of Haiti to the magi and healers of India, there is a specific course of action that is supposed to bring out the soul, the psyche, the supernatural mind, and the true healer within all of us. It's the saint in the cave. It's the blindfold. It's the Indian in the hole covered in darkness until the day he discovers his soul. That is sensory deprivation, and it has a long legacy of miracles attached to it. At the Phoenix Institute and on my own I commit hours of my day to not seeing, hearing, smelling, tasting, or touching. Why? Eight hours of still, quiet, nonsensual deep breathing is known to be the greatest of healers. It's called sleep, in fact, and I believe in the future the sleep process will be a source for incredible solutions in health and healing. The pleasures of the world are fleeting and wonderful, but if you find peace, contentedness, joy, and true forgiveness within, beyond external stimulation, how great a life can you *really* live? This is my rationale, and the lesson, when delivered, absolutely left its impression on my psyche, the nonsensual self. You can visit and go where no man or woman has ever gone. Perhaps it will help the psyche, the soul, and the easy breath, to remember something.

Naturally I've become very interested in sensory deprivation tanks. In health circles, these are the latest craze. Funny enough, I've actually come to understand how incredibly useful it can be to heal the sensual organs. We live most of the time through our senses, so if we live through them, they have an effect on our health. The effect is called "psychosomatic," so I think sensory deprivation and sensory restoration are the great new yin and yang for healing the flesh, the physical frame, the human body, and the servant of the psyche or spirit. For the eyes, nose, and ears I like using Neti pots, osteopathic massages, propolis eye drops, wheat grass, and oil pulling. For the skin, I use Epsom salt baths, saunas, skin brushes, and of course, massages. Today we're going to talk about this yin and yang, sensory deprivation and restoration, and I invite you to think about it yourself.

PREVENTION

"The word doctor comes from the Latin docere, meaning 'to teach.' If someone earns a doctorate, he or she is qualified to teach. If you are a health consultant or a doctor, you are not just a pusher of medicine. There is an unconscious desire in everyone to be taken care of; you, my friend, are the personification of that deep-seated desire, and you're dressed in white. This is why we are going to take a good look today at what it means to be your own doctor, your own health consultant, your own health strategist, your own scientist."

A wise person once told me it would very intelligent of me to study the elements, the basic elements, in order to understand their temperaments and effects on the body. In the future, it will prove very useful indeed. Today we're going to discuss a very powerful concept called *prevention*. For centuries in the East, doctors were not paid when people got sick; they were paid to keep them well. Those doctors were masters, of course, of signs. They were trained to recognize the signs of a body losing its health, and they would prudently go back to their homes, fix a few herbs and things together, maybe collect a few bones or bark from here or there, and return with a decent old-school prescription. That's what they did. They were paid to keep people well. I'd say this is brilliant. Who's got the time to collect bark, bones, roots, and other things like that? Not many people today. Today, people who wish to be well are fighting a losing battle against the unhealthy, unsavory behavior of the herd—a food-addicted herd, a drug-addicted herd, a wine-addicted herd, an entertainment-addicted herd, a television-addicted herd—and the herd dedicates a tremendous amount of trust in the doctor. They very rarely seek out second, third, or fourth opinions from an independent medical professional. When you get sick, it's time to go see the doctor, and the doctor collects good information from your body with scans, questions, blood, urine, and saliva. He does this to show you not what sort of illness you could prevent in the near future, but rather to address the germ, infirmity, or the invisible sufferable condition you already have. When he figures it all out, you say something like, "Thank you, doctor, I just *knew* something was wrong." He smiles and you smile. Then he charges you an unspeakable amount of money, and often you find out there are side effects to the remedy or an undiscovered diagnosis and half the time you're no better than when you came in. That's science these days, science that has come to rely on falsifiability, which means that if you have a respiratory infection, it's the physician's job to prove well beyond a doubt that a healthy, clear lung is not available to you. This a very effective, admirable, and absolutely brilliant strategy that I support wholeheartedly. It is so important.

Let's go back to the ancient Indian doctor in the country. This fellow takes a look at your face, nails, tongue, eyes, listens to your pulse, asks what you've been eating, how you've slept, how you've been breathing, your energy level, your attitude, and other questions. He gathers his information, and what he does next is interesting. He examines what the body has told him, and if the nails were pointing to the heart, if the pulse was pointing to the heart, if the tongue was indicative of the heart, and if the eyes were indicative of the heart, this country doc simply knows what he has to do next—work with the patient's level of knowledge and comfort and impart enough to bring this bad, bad heart back into the beat.

The word *doctor* comes from the Latin *docere*, meaning "to teach." If someone earns a doctorate, he or she is qualified to teach. If you are a health consultant or a doctor, you are not just a pusher of medicine. There is an unconscious desire in everyone to be taken care of; you, my friend, are the personification of that deep-seated desire, and you're dressed in white. This is why we are going to take a good look today at what it means to be your own doctor, your own health consultant, your own health strategist, your own scientist. What can you calibrate on your body right now? Most people don't even know what to look for on the tongue or the eye, let alone gather evidence to discover its cause. Today, right now, I'm fixing to teach you. First, I'm going to tell you four major indicators of good health. If you have all four, chances are very high that you are going to wake up feeling well tomorrow. Here they are.

1. Larger stools. The ancient Chinese believed that death began in the colon. Scottish physician and scientist Dennis Burk once remarked, big stools, small hospitals; small stools, big hospitals. The human body has all the equipment to process energy from foods.

2. Lesser cravings. Really nutritious food that is appropriate for the body's consumption will always trigger a satiety mechanism. That satiety mechanism tells your body, I don't need any more beyond this; thanks, I enjoyed that. That begins to happen to people who eat more raw foods. It can just easily happen to those who eat wholesome cooked foods as well. A person who is addicted to burgers, candy, or hot dogs is usually attempting to digest a certain mineral, element, protein, or substance within that food. However, those

foods are not designed for our digestion. That makes it difficult for the mind, which is tricked into craving these foods for the minerals, proteins, elements, and the like. If the body can get what it actually needs in usable form, it will thrive. More important, it will aid the mind in moving out of its addictions. As a general rule, an overabundance of cravings is a sign of significant digestive malfunction.

3. The urge to be fit. A level of physical fitness is necessary for great health. Physical activity helps to circulate energy through the body. Consider food as energy in; consider exercise as energy out. If energy is blocked in the body, the body's overall energy declines. If you digest food well, you will gain more energy from it. If you are gaining energy from your food by properly digesting it, you will have the urge to run, swim, dance, or just move about. Mental exercises can also be an appropriate outlet for energy.

4. The urge to drink water. When people alter their natural appetites by poisoning their minds and bodies, one of the very first urges to change is thirst. Water is more important than food. You can live for a few months on water before you die; without water, you can live for about one week. Regaining your thirst for water is like regaining your thirst for life.

When you feel sick, start to look at how you are breathing, sleeping, drinking, and your attitude. Look at your diet, exercise, and your environment. Why? Because these fundamentals are pillars of wholeness in health. Right here at the base levels of the holistic health pyramid is where we find those important basic elements of life.

Let's look at breathing. What are we breathing? Well, most of the time we are suffocating and short of breath. The carbon dioxide trapped in our lungs doesn't go anywhere and tends to create an imbalance to an acid-based condition in the body. We also have to ask, what kind of air are we breathing? Is it laden with pollution, or does it have a dynamic balance of nitrogen and oxygen? Hardly anyone these days can say they are breathing perfect-quality air. I suggest indoor plants and filters to bring in nitrogen, oxygen, and carbon dioxide. Now we'll look at hydrogen. Water is the name of the game. The better you hold your water and the more you consume fresh, pure water, the healthier you are going to become. Coffee, alcohol, even herbal teas can rob your body of water and throw off the balance of hydrogen in the body.

Bernard Jensen once put together a very interesting book called *The Chemistry of Man*. In it, he lists the basic elements of the human body and their amounts, and I will read them to you. The average 160-pound man or woman is composed of the following: oxygen, ninety pounds; carbon, thirty-six pounds; hydrogen, fourteen pounds; calcium, three pounds, twelve ounces; nitrogen, three pounds, eight ounces; phosphorous, one pound, four ounces; chlorine, four ounces; sulfur, three to half an ounce; potassium, three ounces; sodium, two to half an ounce; fluorine, two ounces; magnesium, one to twelve ounces; silicon, one-quarter of an ounce; iron, one-sixth of an ounce; and a trace amount of manganese and iodine. I suggest you read *Chemistry of Man* or my book *The Seven Fundamentals of Longevity* for more information.

It's time to ask a funky question: What supplement do I take? How about, what is the best cleanse? Rather, what element is missing?

Am I breathing, hydrated, and sleeping well? What is my weakest health fundamental? How can I get my energy level higher or go to the bathroom? These are clever questions, clever because they strike at the fundamental issues. There are decent answers to every one of these questions, and the answers are meant for you, not for the herd. The answers are always tailored for the individual's need. What's the best supplement the individual can take at night or in the morning? Knowledge. Find out what you need and safely come to a reasonable solution. Calibrate your answers. Check if they can be falsified. Then you will become your own healer. You will become your own scientist. It's simple stuff. If you're uncomfortable with the responsibility, all you have to do is think differently about your own body and its needs. The knowledge is everywhere; all you have to do is look for it.

My Three
Greatest Healers

"Then I met a diabetic who told me he had ceased his insulin shots after six days at Hippocrates. I met a Type 1 diabetic—or former Type 1 diabetic. I had many long conversations with a cancer-free, psoriasis-free, arthritis-free woman who had spent the last eight weeks in the care of Hippocrates Health Institute. And then people dropping weight loss, Lyme's disease, blood pressure. I asked myself, What in God's name is going on here? Then I saw my own nerve-damaged arms, neck, and throat, which I had been told was terminal and permanent, were gone, and then my fair skin stopped burning under the sun and my eyes changed color to a heightened yellow-green. That was two weeks before I dropped six pounds of body weight after a personally historic session of colon hydrotherapy. When I say none of this is bullshit, you know exactly what I mean and where I'm coming from."

Prior to 2007 I had been a spiritual shopper for over three years. That is, I had checked things out, picked up one book on shamanism, another on anthroposophy, took this class on yoga, read that blog on the Kundalini and crystal energy. Spiritual shopping, you know? Looking back today, I'd say my questions were very sincere yet morally unimpressive. I wanted to know what the human body was. If I was something beyond my physical frame, how I could become powerful enough to use this supernatural identity I had sensed? I deeply desired to initiate myself into an understanding of this power. I wanted to know what the "dark knight of the soul" phenomenon from Saint John of the Cross was all about, too. I was wet behind the ears, filled with vigor, and would stop at nothing until I reached my goal. That was a dangerous place to be for a young man, especially one who thought he could rewrite the rules himself.

From September 2007 all the way into November 2007, I learned what the dark knight of the soul was really all about, and hell hath no fury like this poor soul scorned. The floodgates had opened. How corrupted in soul and mind I had become. How unaware and irreverent I was to cause and effect and the goodness that brought me life. My shadow was everywhere. Have you ever been harassed into your own evolution? Has a deep part of yourself ever dragged you across the ground, kicking and screaming, toward personal evolution? It's powerful, and I needed healing. I needed healing so desperately I was willing to not talk for days. I stayed up all night to pray and did very unusual things. No class, no book, no workshop could have ever prepared me for the state of terrific fear in which I would live. I did it alone. Through an act of will and with some expert guidance, I learned to conquer myself. I found that healing that I really needed, and today we are going to talk about three very special and profoundly healing activities that I discovered walking my own path since November 2007.

I'm going to talk about how and where to go when midnight descends on body and soul. I'll say frankly and openly I've earned a few stripes in self-healing, and of course I have many more to go, but what I have to share with you is the very best advice that I, Anthony Canelo, can give. So I hope you give attention to what I'm going to tell you.

First, how did I get through this extreme dissociative entanglement called the "dark knight of the soul"? First, I had to improve my mental acuity. I was told to trace great works of art very slowly for at least one hour per day. I traced the Mona Lisa, Dali, Picasso and many others. It was very healing and a fantastic adjunct to the prayer and meditation. On the suggestion of my friend, Cheryl Stoll, I also wrote a schedule for every day of the week. It was helpful because at the time I was unemployed, broke, alone, traumatized from the events of the prior summer, in poor health, and I had recently moved back to New Jersey. I had to clean out my apartment. I had to clean out everything. I didn't really know what to do with myself, so a schedule helped. The most helpful thing I learned to do was to pray for peace, and it worked. Somehow my prayers were answered in December, when the former owner of The Phoenix Institute, Charles Walters, offered me the chance to run his beloved business. I think he made a very good decision. Where fear had once been now lived impregnable strength and courage. Where corruption and abuse had lived, now there was power and respect. Where naiveté had been, skepticism, boldness, and pioneering curiosity now lived, and I was just finally beginning to get in touch with my deep sorrows. I had become a man. In December my family celebrated the year. I was busy learning my craft and helping people with their footbaths, colon cleanses, and massages.

Then I visited the Hippocrates Health Institute in West Palm Beach, Florida. You know what made an impression on me right from the beginning? The old man who walked beside me in the food aisle said that he had just tossed his wheelchair in the dumpster. Then I saw another old man do the same, and the next day these old men were walking faster, with brighter smiles and rosier skin. Then I met a diabetic who told me he had ceased his insulin shots after six days at Hippocrates. I met a Type 1 diabetic—or former Type 1 diabetic. I had many long conversations with a cancer-free, psoriasis-free, arthritis-free woman who had spent the last eight weeks in the care of Hippocrates Health Institute. and then people dropping weight loss, Lyme's disease, blood pressure. I asked myself, *What in God's name is going on here?* Then I saw my own nerve-damaged arms, neck, and throat, which I had been told was terminal and permanent, were gone, and then my fair skin stopped burning under the sun and my eyes changed color to a heightened yellow-green. That was two weeks before I dropped six pounds of body weight after a personally historic session of colon hydrotherapy. When I say none of this is bullshit, you know exactly what I mean and where I'm coming from.

The Hippocrates Health Institute was and is the inspired vision of Ann Wigmore. The institute promotes a deeper connection to nature through raw living foods, fresh air and exercise, clean water, and a healthy attitude. That means, to those of you who are the audience of the Revival, that they had and still do have a deeper understanding of their connection to nature than most. When it comes to the average day, it's a very genius routine of sprout juices, vegetables, wheat grass, workshops, lectures, and sunshine. In no uncertain terms, Hippocrates is a remarkable oasis in the South Florida environment. When I left, I had grown prodigiously. I had fasted, cleaned out, swum forty laps in their mineral pool every day, and read vociferously. I was on fire, and then I came home. Within two days I had built a rather large indoor garden completely by myself. My mind was bursting with an energy that forced me to begin writing. You know, I haven't stopped. To be honest, I'm still on fire. I don't follow the raw living food, vegan Hippocrates diet completely. I found that my body required additional forms of energy. What really got the creative juices going? What healed my body and freshened my mind and spirit? Hippocrates Health Institute was the first great healer, and they got the ball rolling. With the knowledge I gained, I ended up helping hundreds of people.

Once I had a client named Vince, and Vince was part of a large Puerto Rican family. He lived in a tightly knit community. I showed him everything I had learned at Hippocrates: how to sprout your vegetable seeds and beans and why you should; how to blend green protein juices and smoothies; Epsom salt and ginger baths; and supplementing with vitamin B_{12}, magnesium, vitamin C, wheat grass, and blue-green algae. He ended up losing thirty pounds, but I think all that energy went right to his heart and brain, because he began to send me each member of his family. To my genuine surprise, they really paid attention. Most of them healed very nicely. That was when Vince brought it back to West Patterson and Union, New Jersey. Since then, he's helped scores or maybe hundreds of people as well. I'm very happy and very proud to have planted that first seed and watched it sprout.

The next great healer in my life was a school, a school that was bold enough to show me how small I was and challenged me to be great. This special school would become the seminal influence of my life—influential, informative, groundbreaking, original. The greatest healing force I had ever found, I found in the most stark and contrasting of ways. Her name is J. Z. Knight, and his name is Ramtha, the Enlightened One. The school is called Ramtha School of Enlightenment, or RSE for short, and if you do a little "research" on the Internet you will find an ocean of controversy. Yet whatever controversy you find in the public eye is often flattery waiting in disguise. What do they know? If the school were measured by the productivity, reputations, gentility, upright characters, genius, and abilities of its student body, rather than by its highly unorthodox teacher, they are surely the unheralded fruits to the great tree that is Ramtha School, so I'm proud to be a part of the great work.

How did I find out about this school all the way up here in New Jersey? During October 2007 I saw three words pop up in my mind when I logged onto Amazon.com: *The White Book*. I bought it, loved it, and kept reading. Then I watched a DVD that I'd personally give as my sole recommendation to anyone interested in this school, *Create Your Day*, which happens to be the sequel to the very famous independent film *What the Bleep Do We Know!?* The Ramtha School has been around for forty years, published hundreds if not thousands of CDs and books, and helped to heal the minds, bodies, and spirits of thousands. I've seen people correct major scoliosis with simple breathing and dedicated concentration.

Another student from the school writes that Ramtha's teachings are neither a new religion nor the building blocks of a new church. His teachings are a system of thought that contains within its approach to reality the elements and mechanisms that allow the individual to engage Ramtha's philosophy and verify and experience its content firsthand. In other words, this unique aspect of the teachings allows the philosophy or concepts of reality to be experienced and become instead wisdom about the nature of reality. Ramtha's system of thought and disciplines are direct, pure, and uncomplex. They resemble sacred knowledge practiced by the ancient mystery schools of Greece, Egypt, and the Middle East as well as the ancient Gnostic schools of the Middle East and Europe. This important characteristic helps to distinguish Ramtha's teachings from traditional philosophical schools of the Western world.

So what do they give? An original take on humanity's most fundamental question: Who am I? Why am I? How am I, and what will I do with this knowledge? Rich and valuable interpretations of quantum physics, neurology, human history, social psychology, and the nature of spirit and soul are revealed and reveled in the most poetic and concise form. Ramtha can talk the talk. I don't think I know anyone with a larger vocabulary. To be sure, he can walk the talk just as easily. He's a pleasure to be with in person. When it comes to the mind, body, spirit dynamic, I've found that RSE is very helpful and very worthwhile. Many nights of the week I sit down to hot tea and play my favorite albums before I sleep: "The Legacy Teachings," "The Mystery of the Invisible," or "Gardening for Transmutation." Whereas Hippocrates Health Institute helped me experience a connection to nature, Ramtha gave me his own expert guidance on how to find it.

Last, but definitely not least, is the wonderful practice of the five rhythms. Gabrielle Roth once said it takes discipline to be a free spirit. Put the body in motion, and the psyche will heal itself. One day, while working at Esalen, Ms. Roth decided to turn on some music, take off her shoes, stop talking, stop pretending, and just start moving, and she has helped people get to the same place in so many ways. The five rhythms is a turn-yourself-inside-out, shoeless, explanation-less free movement, a totally and utterly unstructured royal throwdown of the human spirit. Call it a tribal dance if you want, but it is happening all over the world and goes on every night of the week in Manhattan, New York City. It's so nice to dance to great music alone in our rooms, cooped up nicely in our pretty worlds, and sometimes it's nice to do the same with one hundred other people to impressive music on the top floor of a New York City building on a Friday or Saturday night for two hours.

Has it healed me? Oh, you had better start believing it now. Pack your bags with clothing you plan to sweat through, bring a lot of water, and join the five rhythms class closest to you. Just get in touch with that primeval, simple, witch doctor soul of yours. I'm there all the time. After the Hippocrates Health experience and Ramtha's teachings I come to celebrate my connection to nature with five rhythms. Hippocrates, RSE, and five rhythms are my personal treasures. They are worth more to me than almost anything. Thank you for listening, my friends, and have a productive, enlightening, exciting rest of your day.

GREATEST GOOD,
LEAST EFFORT

"I have mentioned in early readings that these Will to Live Centers could help specifically address the most preventable causes of death in the United States of America. Think of my common sense questions."

If you want to kick an addiction, I suggest you try to get really good at doing the opposite of your addiction. In fact, exercise is the most popular and effective way to quit smoking cigarettes. The best way to kick alcohol is to clean your liver and blood and exercise. To best way to handle food addiction is to fast or eat healthy foods that satisfy the body. The best way to kick laziness is to simply breathe and then get out and start walking. Slowness is the remedy for busyness. Moderation is an outstanding cure for obsession. If you don't understand yourself as a man, there's an option to study your opposite in a woman and vice versa. Suppose you do not understand the human body at all. I would suggest that you study its opposite, its symbiote: the tree. The roots of the tree could liken to the bowel, the gut. The trunk of the tree is the liver, blood, and pancreas. The senses could be the flowers. The mind, the soul. The ghost in the machine might liken to sunshine. If you struggle to achieve peak performance, you could think of the body as a sound system. The master control unit is the liver, blood, or bowel. The CD, cassette, or iPod is the heart, pancreas, thyroid, and adrenals. The microphone and speakers are the neurotransmitters, senses, nervous system, brain, and spine. Acoustics are exercise and self-control.

Master volume is breath and self-control. Genre of music could be ethical or spiritual principle.

If you struggle with figuring out why you should take care of your body, think of it as an automobile. If you don't take care of the engine, you won't be driving anywhere to be on vacation. Sometimes the body can be likened to a river, because every moment is a unique orchestration of impulses and chemistry. You can call the body a cave because it is created from the most primeval elements of nature, and yet there's a glimmer of light that always comes through the head. You can call the body a bridge because it is a sovereign vehicle, and using it, you're able to connect your own nature to nature. You can remember Samuel Thompson, the first American herbalist, who said that the body was like a furnace and requests long-burning fuel, space, and the occasional clearing of the chimneys.

Let's not forget the holistic health pyramid and the seven fundamentals of health, breathing, sleeping, drinking, attitude, exercise, eating, and a connection to nature. You see, the body is really one vast ecosystem and within it there are simpler, tinier ecosystems. A wise person once wrote that it takes more energy to die than to live. It helps to see the body in a brand-new light sometimes, because the simple truth is that we live in an unhealthy culture. According to *Forbes* magazine and myself, there are seven preventable causes of death in the United States: smoking, alcohol, drugs, sexually transmitted diseases, lack of exercise and nutrition, lack of hygiene, and a toxic lifestyle. These are potholes, river dams, blowouts, dynamite, and chain saws. They are the top seven biggest problems in our culture. This is why I think we should organize Will To Live Centers all over the country. I have mentioned in early readings that these Will to Live Centers could help specifically address the most preventable causes of death in the United States of America. Think of my common sense questions:

1. What is the smallest thing you can do that would help create the largest shift in your life?

2. What is the largest thing you can do that would create the most insignificant shift in your life?

3. Which unhealthy habit could you cease that would yield the smallest real effect on your life?

4. What is the simplest, smallest thing you could stop doing that would bring on the most tremendously powerful impact for the good in your own life?

I wrote a book called *Self-Determination* detailing how one can master these seven addictions. For smoking, vitamins like nonmethylated B_{12}, liquorice, lobelia, and niacinamide can help reduce cravings. Feverfew, cayenne pepper, and catnip can help you overcome headaches from withdrawal. Coconut oil and vitamin B_{12} can help an alcoholic overcoming the sickness of withdrawal. I thought of writing this book because I prefer to think in terms of the least-effort greatest good, and I hope that you're able to see it too. Addiction is a rough road. It's time to look at your body another way. Likewise, it's time to look at the body of humanity a little differently. Another perspective. That is why we're here, ladies and gentlemen.

BUILDING THE
NATURE PYRAMID

"That's my dream, baby."

The goal of a great civilization is to build toward a connection to nature. If anyone got it right the first time, it was the Egyptians. Right from the start, the Egyptians displayed a very complete knowledge of dental care, hygiene, plant medicines, brain surgery, and a metaphysical science that was quantum leaps ahead of its time. Of course, as we all know, they began building the fiery forms. The lost civilization of the Mayans and the Incas were likewise far ahead of their time, showing profound skill in construction, complex mathematics, and the study of the stars. They were one of the first civilizations of the Americas, and somehow they too began building the fiery forms. In fact, the fiery forms were also built in North America. Anyone who has ever visited Pyramid State Park in Illinois would know. Let's not forget about the Chinese with their complete system of physical, environmental, and energy medicine and their fiery forms, or the ancient Okinawans who built their pyramids where the ocean floor now sits. Fascinating, isn't it? Out of the blue the simultaneous miracle of civilization comes complete with organizing and physiological principles that university professors still spend their days drooling over.

So what's my point? If you believe that a great civilization is destined for a direct course toward harmony with the natural world, not only have we regressed, we have ignored the primeval tools of success that made these arcane cultures great. So, what is the pyramid? The pyramid was a central part of ancient life. A pyramid, or pyra-mid, literally translates to "fire in the middle." At the top of a true fiery form is a perfect right angle. Isn't it so incredible how every single great civilization all over the world and perhaps even in Antarctica built its fiery forms with the same right angle? Wow, what an inconvenience to debunkers who are out there. By this time you might be thinking, "I've heard of sacred geometry, why are you teasing us with these questions?" Well, here is why, my friends. I have a dream. It is a dream deeply rooted in the dreams of Ahkmenrah and Imhotep. I have a dream that one day we will begin to restore our sacred connection to nature, and in doing so, we will build the most beautiful, productive, provocative, healing, balancing, and nurturing holistic health pyramid hospitals. Brothers and sisters, I have a dream that one day these pyramid hospitals will cover the land and reset our primary, our sacred connection to nature. That's my dream, baby; that's my dream. In New Jersey at The Phoenix Institute of Holistic Health, I have a dear guest named Gerard who comes in for his weekly foot baths. Since I introduced him to the seven fundamentals of longevity—breathing, sleeping, hydration, attitude, nutrition, fitness and nature—and since I mentioned to him my plan to build these seven-leveled hospitals all over the world, he has without fail, during every single foot bath, found an appropriate point in the conversation to say to me "and then you gon' build that pyramid." It's a great running joke, but he and I will one day be laughing much, much harder once he starts getting foot baths on the third floor of my holistic health pyramid next to the pure water bar, juice bar, and bath house. That would be above the dark floor, which will be above the hermetically sealed gardens with hedonic air quality…but I digress.

The pyramids are relics of a golden era of pure understanding, and that understanding is the understanding of the natural world. The term "sacred geometry" is much older than "the new age." Sacred geometry is real. Many of you remember the globed-shaped tomato baskets they used to sell in the sixties. Those are a great example of the power of sacred geometry. Those tomatoes would not grow in containers of any other shape—not a cube or a pentagon. They need curves to grow, and many of you have heard of the golden ratio. That's the ratio present in nearly all of life. The arm-to-wing spans, stamen-to-stalk, curve of a seashell, arms of the galaxy—everything is built with mathematical precision. Sacred math creates sacred geometry, and sacred geometry is built into the natural world. It isn't new age. Pythagoras really had it figured out, and likewise Picasso, da Vinci, and Fibonacci. Studies have shown that men and women with sacred geometric facial bone ratios appear to have perfect teeth and appear to be more attractive than the "lesser aligned." That's a horrible sounding word, but this is deep science, the science of a sacred mathematics. Everything has a number, vibration, and power, even our thoughts. As a few of you know, the frequency consciousness pyramid of the Ramtha School of Enlightenment is what helped to inspire me to create my own pyramid. That seven-level frequency pyramid—Hertzian body, infrared body, light body, ultraviolent blue body, x-ray body, gamma body, and infinite unknown body—is far ahead of its time. It might help you to understand how quantum physics, the study of light particles, will lead us to the new science of tomorrow, the ultraviolet physics.

Talk about food for thought, huh? What I've done is create a concept called "the holistic health pyramid" that reflects the strategic unfolding of your connection to nature. It begins with the breath, because without breath you have death. Next on the order is sleep, because sleeping is healing; there is no greater medicine. Most of us were not taught that, with age, melatonin naturally decreases, so the older you get the more restoration and healing you will need at night. That's why maximizing your quality of rest is so important. Level three is drinking, because without hydration your health care strategy does not hold water. Attitude is the fourth fundamental, and this represents the higher of chain of command for fitness, nutrition, and health environment. All of this is very real and based on the metabolic function of the body. If your understanding of health and wellness begins with exercise and ends with a healthier diet, you're playing a zero sum game, and you know it. This is the connection to nature you've been looking for. It's about health. It's my message, my books, my writing, and my whole life.

Now it will probably be a while before they start building the first pyra-hospital, but I've had the opportunity to imagine what life would be like in harmony with sacred mathematics and geometry. I created two things I'd like to share. Did you know that in the center of the great pyramid in Egypt fruit does not spoil, the air is still, carcasses do not decay, and the temperature is a constant 68 degrees Fahrenheit? It's a remarkable thing and perhaps the reason why the pyramid is known as a wonder of the world. Who could have built something as stunning as the Pyramid of Giza? It would take your local township well over twenty years. You know what I tell them? Better late than never. I created the bamboo pyramid with instructions in my book *Sleep the Great Medicine* because I want people to comprehend the real power behind the fiery form. You simply purchase six-foot or eight-foot bamboo poles, rubber bands, a measuring tape, perhaps a few crystals here or there, and follow instructions. The total would cost maybe fifty dollars, which is a deal if you start looking up the cost for personalized wooden pyramids elsewhere.

I also came up with a new idea I call the sacred geometric yoga, and this involves one or more persons making squares, circles, or pyramids on their yoga mats and meditating in those positions. Imagine that you're sitting cross-legged, back to back, man and woman, hands on knees. That's a pyramid with a masculine positive charge and a feminine negative charge and something you could try at home. There is so much one can do with sacred math and the holistic health pyramid. One day someone will have enough courage to start their sacred geometric civilization, and perhaps when they begin building, they will figure out the best structure for the "temples" of wellness and good health. That day, if it should come, someone will be reading someone else's plans. This is my manifesto, my plan, my big dream. Until that day, those big dreams and big plans are safely locked away. It is my hope that I may be of some use, although only time will tell. Thank you.

www.ingramcontent.com/pod-product-compliance
Lightning Source LLC
Chambersburg PA
CBHW030443290526
45786CB00001B/415

* 9 7 8 1 4 9 6 0 7 8 9 6 4 *